Colour **Aids**

KU-154-495

Infectious Diseases

A.P. Ball FRCPEd
Infectious Diseases Unit
Cameron Hospital
Windygates
Fife
Scotland

J.A. Gray FRCPEd
Infectious Diseases Unit
City Hospital
Edinburgh
Scotland

Churchill Livingstone

EDINBURGH LONDON MELBOURNE AND NEW YORK 1984

Acknowledgements

The authors gratefully acknowledge the kind permission of the following colleagues and others, to reproduce photographs from their collections:

Dr E. Edmond (Fig. 12), Dr R. Hume (Figs 33, 57, 58), Dr R. Fothergill (Figs 35, 36, 37, 38, 39, 93), Dr M. McDonald (Figs 55, 56), Dr A.C. Scott (Fig. 94), Dr J.A. Innes (Fig. 120) and Abbott Laboratories Ltd (Figs 78, 79).

Special thanks are due to the Medical Photography Department, Victoria Hospital, Kirkcaldy, Fife, and to Mrs E. Shields and Mrs M. Horne for invaluable secretarial assistance.

Contents

1 | Measles (1)

Aetiology

Measles virus, a single serotype paramyxovirus.

Incidence

Common in pre-school and junior schoolchildren, notably in the last few months of the year. The pattern is usually sporadic or sub-epidemic but explosive outbreaks can occur if measles virus is introduced to previously unexposed communities.

Pathogenesis

Case-to-case spread follows airborne droplet transmission from the respiratory tract of patients with active measles. There is no other reservoir of infection. Invasion of the upper respiratory tract and conjunctivae is followed by multiplication in lymphoid tissues and viraemia. Histological appearances are characterised by mononuclear reaction with giant cells and endothelial proliferation. Lesions are present in skin (rash), mucous membranes (Koplik's spots), lungs, gut and lymphoid tissue.

Clinical features

The incubation period of 2 wk is followed by an upper respiratory catarrhal prodromal phase, with Koplik's spots on buccal mucosa (Fig. 1) accompanied by conjunctivitis, otitis media and rhinitis (Fig. 2). This is followed 24–48 h later by a dusky red rash, commencing on the face and spreading peripherally via the trunk (Figs 3, 4 & 5). Uncomplicated measles lasts for 7–10 d. The rash fades leaving staining — brown macules with fine desquamation — which can persist for up to 3 wk (Fig. 6).

Complications

1. Secondary bacterial otitis media, bronchopneumonia and purulent conjunctivitis: usually caused by pneumococci and *Haemophilus influenzae*, but also by *Staphylococcus aureus*.
2. Obstructive laryngitis and dysentery: both associated with childhood and infant malnutrition in developing countries.

INFECTIOUS DISEASES

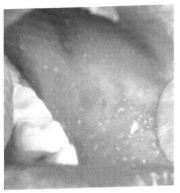

Fig. 1 Koplik's spots on buccal mucosa.

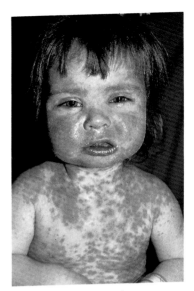

Fig. 2 Morbilliform rash, conjunctivitis and rhinitis.

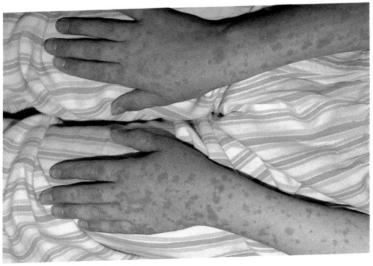

Fig. 3 Detail of measles rash.

Measles (2)

**Compli-
cations**
(contd)

3. Appendicitis: increased incidence in measles.
4. Giant cell pneumonitis: a rare diffuse pulmonary infiltration causing respiratory failure.
5. Allergic encephalomyelitis: onset 1–2 wk after measles. Incidence 1 : 6000 cases.
6. Sub-acute sclerosing panencephalitis: reactivation of latent virus within brain after 5–7 yr causing fatal encephalitis. Death is inevitable within 6–12 mth. Incidence 1 : 1 000 000 cases.
7. Atypical measles: hyperpyrexia, vesicular rash and pneumonia. Usually seen in adults who received inactivated vaccine in the 1960s.

Treatment

Symptomatic. Erythromycin (30 mg kg/d) or cloxacillin–amoxycillin combination are effective for bacterial complications. There is no effective antiviral therapy for acute complications such as pneumonitis. Steroids are of marginal value in allergic encephalitis. Isoprinosine may temporarily arrest progression of sclerosing panencephalitis but does not affect eventual fatal outcome.

Prevention

Notifiable: hospitalised cases must be isolated
1. *Active immunisation:* attenuated vaccine gives 97% seroconversion and long term immunity. About 3% of vaccinees develop a mild febrile reaction.
2. *Passive immunisation:* human normal immunoglobulin protects if given within 72 h of exposure.

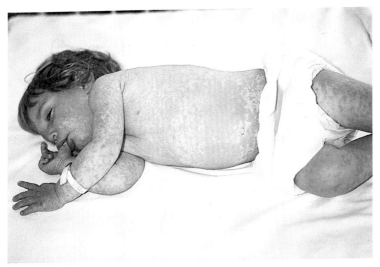

Fig. 4 Fully developed measles rash.

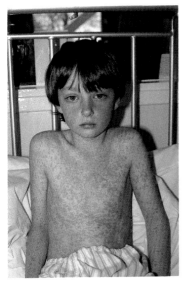

Fig. 5 Fully developed measles rash.

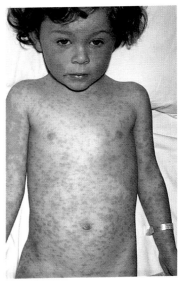

Fig. 6 Post-measles staining.

2 | Rubella

Aetiology

Rubella virus, a single serotype togavirus.

Incidence

Common in schoolchildren with occasional epidemic fluctuations.

Pathogenesis

Case-to-case airborne droplet transmission from the respiratory tract of active cases. Invasion by the upper respiratory tract is followed by dissemination to skin, conjunctivae and mucous membranes and a resultant mild mononuclear reaction and proliferative hyperplasia in lymph nodes. Lesions occur in the skin, lymphoid tissue, conjunctivae.

Clinical features

The incubation period of $2\frac{1}{2}$–3 wk is followed by mild upper respiratory catarrh, conjunctival suffusion and, within 24–48 h, a discrete maculopapular generalised rash (Figs 7–10). Lymphadenopathy is prominent, notably of suboccipital and postauricular groups. Systemic upset is minimal. The rash may last 5 d but is often fleeting and fades without staining or desquamation. Rubella is diagnosed by the haemagglutination–inhibition and IgM tests.

Complications

1. Immune complex arthritis: typically affecting small joints, develops in 10% of women.
2. Allergic encephalomyelitis: commences 10–14 d after rubella. Incidence 1 : 6000.
3. Purpura: caused by thrombocytopenia and vascular defects (rare).
4. Congenital rubella syndrome (p. 7).

Treatment

Symptomatic. Non-steroidal anti-inflammatory agents may be required for rubella arthritis.

Prevention

Not notifiable: hospitalised cases must be isolated. Live attenuated rubella vaccines (Cendehill and RA27/3 strains) give high level protection.

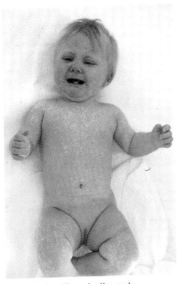

Fig. 7 Infantile rubella rash.

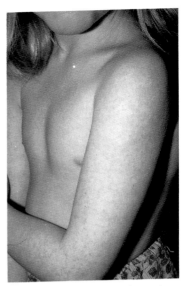

Fig. 8 Discrete pink macular rash.

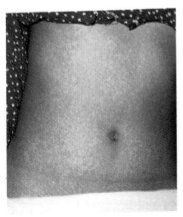

Fig. 9 Profuse rash in adult.

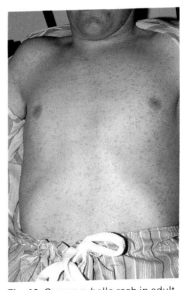

Fig. 10 Sparse rubella rash in adult.

3 | Congenital Rubella Syndrome (CRS)

Aetiology

Rubella virus (p. 5).

Incidence

Affects up to 40% of fetuses exposed to maternal rubella during first trimester. About 60 cases per year in the UK despite prevention programme.

Pathogenesis

Follows transplacental fetal infection by rubella virus. Highest risk between 6–8 wk gestation but possible risk up to 16–18 wk. Widespread fetal involvement includes persistent infection of liver, heart, CNS, lungs, pancreas and long bones. Neonatal jaundice and purpura are often present. Dysorganogenesis results in major ophthalmic, cardiac, auditory and neurological abnormalities in 10% of affected pregnancies.

Clinical features

Severe CRS may include: pulmonary stenosis, PDA (common), coarction and VSD (rare) (Fig. 11); microphathalmia, cataract (Fig. 12) and retinitis; sensorineural deafness and microcephaly. Severe mental deficiency is uncommon. The extended syndrome may include purpura, anaemia, metaphyseal dysplasia, hepatitis, myocarditis, pneumonitis and low birth weight.

Treatment

Non-immune mothers who develop clinical or serological evidence of rubella in early pregnancy (< 15 wk) are offered therapeutic abortion. Rubella immune globulin does not prevent congenital rubella.

Prevention

Immunisation programme in UK aims to immunise all 11–13-year-old girls using Cendehill and RA27/3 live-attenuated vaccines. Non-immune pregnant women exposed to rubella who do not seroconvert must be immunised in the immediate puerperium.

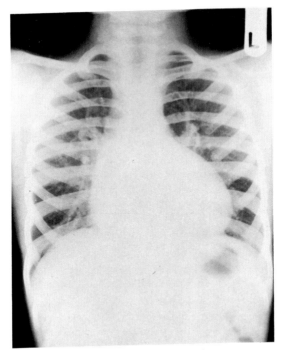

Fig. 11 Congenital ventricular septal defect.

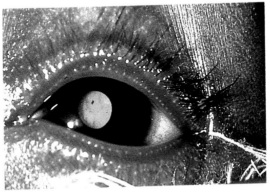

Fig. 12 Congenital rubella cataract.

4 | Mumps

Aetiology

Mumps virus, a single serotype paramyxovirus.

Incidence

All ages may be affected; commoner in children over 1 yr. Subclinical infection is common. World-wide distribution. Seven year cycles, clustering in spring and winter.

Pathogenesis

Moderately infectious: spreads by airborne droplet transmission from active cases. This is followed by viraemia and glandular involvement. Salivary glands: interstitial oedema and lymphocyte invasion. Testes: oedema, perivascular lymphocyte invasion, focal haemorrhage, destruction of germinal epithelium and tubular plugging. The CNS, pancreas, ovaries, breasts, thyroid and joints are less frequently involved.

Clinical features

The incubation period of 14–18 d is followed by a generalised febrile illness, sometimes associated with convulsions in small children. Tender parotid or submandibular gland swelling (Figs 13 & 14), bilateral in 70%, surrounded by oedema, lasts for a few days. Meningeal irritation is common. Mumps virus is easily cultured from saliva or CSF. Paired sera show an antibody titre rise.

Complications

1. Orchitis in 20% of postpubertal males (Fig. 15). Bilateral orchitis may result in subfertility.
2. Lymphocytic meningitis (frequent).
3. Postinfectious encephalitis, pancreatitis, oophoritis and thyroiditis are all rare. Large joint arthritis occurs infrequently.

Treatment

Symptomatic. Prednisolone may relieve orchitis.

Prevention

In some countries live attenuated mumps vaccine is given with measles and rubella vaccine in second year of life.

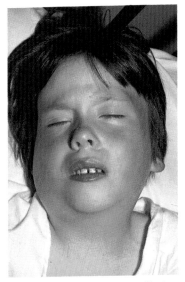

Fig. 13 Parotid and submandibular gland swelling.

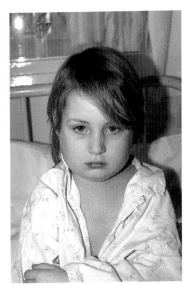

Fig. 14 Mumps parotitis.

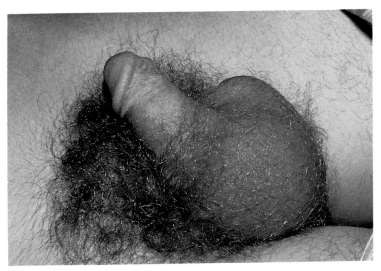

Fig. 15 Mumps orchitis.

5 | Chickenpox (1)

Aetiology

Varicella-zoster virus: a DNA containing herpes virus. Synonyms: varicella, herpes zoster.

Incidence

World-wide distribution: common in children after 9 mth, with clusters in winter and early spring. Less common but more severe in adults. Congenital and neonatal chickenpox are rare.

Pathogenesis

Highly infectious: spreads by airborne droplet transmission from active cases of chickenpox (and shingles). Histologically identical skin lesions occur in the middle and deep epidermis in both chickenpox and shingles. Cell damage produces oedema which forms clear vesicle fluid. This transforms into a cloudy pustule after WBC invade and then a scab which separates leaving a fine papery scar. The base of the lesion contains intranuclear inclusions and multinucleate giant cells. An enanthem (mucosal rash) is common. Chickenpox may cause a haemorrhagic, oedematous, necrotic pneumonia and pleurisy, often more severe in immunocompromised patients. Miliary calcification may follow. Encephalitis is unusual.
Keratitis and corneal ulcers are seen less often than with H.simplex infection. Haemorrhagic chickenpox results from thrombocytopenia and consumption coagulopathy.

Clinical features

The incubation period is about 2 wk (range 7–23 d). Influenza-like symptoms may precede the rash in adults but in children the rash (Figs 16 & 17) starts first, often with little fever. Each spot starts as a macule then progresses through vesicular, pustular and crusting stages unless aborted by antiviral agents. Crops of spots occur every day or two (Fig. 18). The scalp, face, trunk and hollows of the body are more affected than the limbs and prominences. The rash is accompanied by an enanthem (Figs 16 & 19) and may be very sparse or, notably in immunocompromised patients,

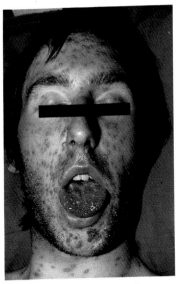

Fig. 16 Facial exanthem and enanthem on tongue.

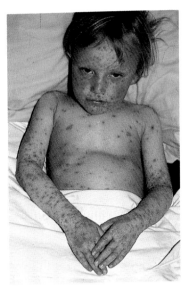

Fig. 17 Distribution in eczematous child (atypical).

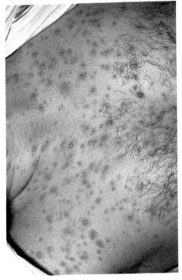

Fig. 18 Crops of papules, vesicles and pustules.

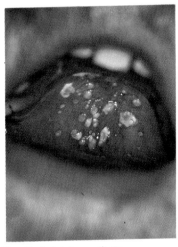

Fig. 19 Palatal enanthem.

5 | Chickenpox (2)

Clinical features (contd)

profuse (Fig. 20). The uncomplicated illness lasts about 7 d. Diagnosis is confirmed by virus isolation from vesicle fluid and rising antibody titres.

Complications

Secondary bacterial infection of the spots causes septic lesions or progresses to varicella gangrenosa (Fig. 21). Neonates, the elderly or immunodeficient patients may develop severe pneumonia (Figs 22 & 23). A rare encephalopathy usually causes mild, transient cerebellar signs but can be fatal.

Treatment

Largely symptomatic. Secondary skin sepsis, usually caused by staphylococci or streptococci, may require oral erythromycin treatment. Intravenous acyclovir, a nucleoside antiviral agent, is often highly effective in severely ill neonates or the immunosuppressed.

Prevention

Patients should be isolated from non-immune or immunocompromised patients. Zoster immune globulin may prevent disease in vulnerable contacts. No live vaccine is yet available.

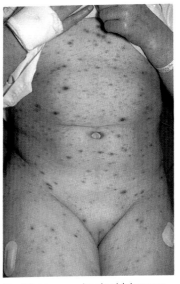

Fig. 20 Haemorrhagic chickenpox in acute leukaemia.

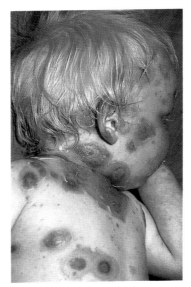

Fig. 21 Varicella gangrenosa.

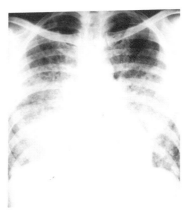

Fig. 22 Acute chickenpox pneumonia.

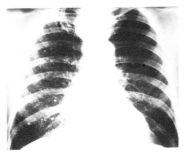

Fig. 23 Chickenpox pneumonia: late calcification.

6 | Herpes Zoster (Shingles) (1)

Aetiology

The varicella-zoster (V-Z) virus: a DNA containing herpes virus.

Incidence

World-wide distribution (as chickenpox) but no seasonal variation. Commoner in the elderly.

Pathogenesis

Skin lesions in H.zoster are histologically identical to chickenpox but follow sensory cranial or peripheral nerve root distributions with inflammation and necrosis of ganglion cells. Motor cells are infrequently affected. Widespread lesions occur in the immunocompromised. V-Z virus is neurotropic, often lying dormant in CNS tissue for many years after childhood chickenpox, until reactivated. Reactivation can complicate immunosuppression due to malignancy, corticosteroid and cytotoxic drugs or radiotherapy but such precipitants are usually absent. Shingles is less infectious than chickenpox.

Clinical features

Burning pain or paraesthesia in the affected dermatome are the usual presenting features. Pain can be mild or severe and of short or long duration, sometimes being replaced by protracted post-herpetic neuralgia. A day or so after the pain starts, skin lesions appear, confined to the affected dermatome with evolution from macule, through vesicle, pustule, crust and scar as in chickenpox. Vesiculopustular lesions often coalesce. A girdle-like eruption following a unilateral thoracic dermatome is the commonest manifestation (Figs 24, 25 & 29), but any sensory nerve can be affected, e.g. supraclavicular nerves (Fig. 28). Sacral shingles may interfere with bladder and bowel function.

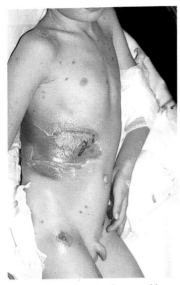

Fig. 24 Herpes zoster (unusual in children).

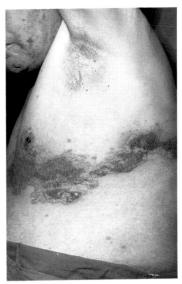

Fig. 25 Fully developed thoracic zoster: limited to single dermatome.

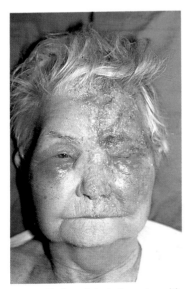

Fig. 26 Early ophthalmic zoster with secondary infection.

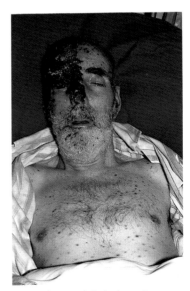

Fig. 27 Late ophthalmic zoster: generalised rash in leukaemia.

Clinical features (contd)

Limb girdle or peripheral limb involvement may be associated with mixed motor and sensory disturbance. Mixed motor and sensory involvement is also seen in the rare Ramsay–Hunt syndrome ('geniculate herpes' — Fig. 30) comprising pain in the middle ear, vesicles on the external auditory meatus, auricle and pharynx with facial palsy and loss of taste. Any branch of the trigeminal nerve may be affected, but herpes zoster ophthalmicus is commonest (Figs 26 & 27). When the nasociliary branch is involved, corneal damage may result. Virus may be grown on tissue culture from the skin lesions. Antibody titres rise during the illness in most patients.

Compli-cations

Secondary bacterial infection may occur. In immunocompromised patients extensive disseminated skin lesions can resemble chickenpox. Pneumonia and meningoencephalitis are uncommon.

Treatment

Analgesics are usually required. Secondary staphylococcal or streptococcal infection responds to oral erythromycin. 5–40% idoxuridine in demethylsulphoxide (DMSO) applied to skin lesions in the first week can abort progression. Oral acyclovir is also effective. Generalised chickenpox complicating shingles may require i.v. acyclovir. H. zoster ophthalmicus usually requires ocular chloramphenicol, homatropine and acyclovir and sometimes corticosteroids.

Prevention

Once acquired, V-Z virus may erupt as shingles at any time. Patients with overt infection should be isolated.

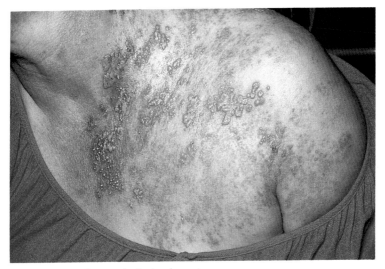

Fig. 28 Zoster of supraclavicular dermatomes.

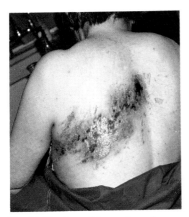

Fig. 29 Healing of thoracic zoster.

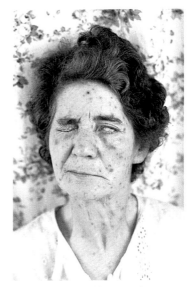

Fig. 30 Ramsay–Hunt syndrome: facial palsy.

Herpes Simplex Infections (1)

Aetiology

Two DNA-containing viruses, distinguishable epidemiologically, clinically and serologically as Herpes simplex types 1 and 2 (HSV-1 and HSV-2). Synonyms: Herpesvirus hominis I/II.

Incidence

Primary HSV-1 infection is usually acquired in infancy by the airborne droplet route. Congenital infection with HSV-1 is rare. Congenital HSV-2 disease may occur but is less common than perinatal infection acquired from the maternal birth canal. Most HSV-2 infection in adults is sexually acquired especially by homosexuals and the promiscuous.

Pathogenesis

Non-immunes are vulnerable to virus shed from the skin and mucosae of active cases over several days. HSV-1 usually affects the mucocutaneous junctions of lips and nose and HSV-2 the genitalia. Virus replication in the epithelium or mucosae causes inflammation, cell lysis and thin walled vesicles. After primary infection HSV-1 and HSV-2 migrate to nerves where they lie dormant. Reactivation may be precipitated by bacterial infection (herpes febrilis), sunlight, menstruation and immunosuppression.

Clinical features

Primary HSV-1 stomatitis consists of painful ulcerating vesicles on the lips, anterior buccal mucosa and nares (Figs 31 & 32). Dendritic corneal ulcers can cause blindness and are more common in HSV-1 than HSV-2 infections. Congenital HSV-1 or HSV-2 infection (Fig. 33) causes jaundice, thombocytopenia, hepatosplenomegaly, rashes, encephalopathy and choroidoretinitis. In eczematous patients HSV-1 infection may be widespread (Kaposi's varicelliform eruption, eczema herpeticum Fig. 34).

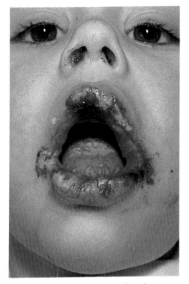

Fig. 31 Primary herpes simplex stomatitis.

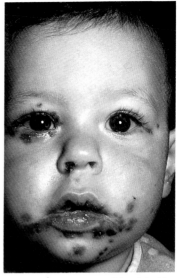

Fig. 32 Primary stomatitis with skin, nasal and periocular involvement.

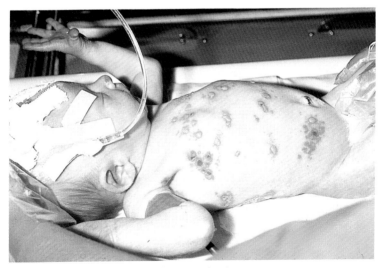

Fig. 33 Congenital disseminated Herpes simplex.

Herpes Simplex Infections (2)

Clinical features (contd)

Primary HSV-2 infection usually affects the genitalia or anus with clusters of painful vesicles lasting for 10 d (Fig. 36). Health care workers may be infected on the fingers, resulting in herpetic whitlow (Fig. 35). HSV-1 encephalitis may complicate neonatal, primary or asymptomatic reactivation of virus with focal CNS signs, confusion and coma. CSF is often normal but brain scan shows focal disease.

Virus can be isolated from the infected mouth, anus and genitals and, in encephalitis, from brain biopsy but usually not from CSF. Serology is diagnostic in primary infections but is of little value during reactivations or encephalitis.

Treatment

Iodine mouthwashes are valuable in stomatitis. Local acyclovir or idoxuridine (IDU) is useful for ocular and skin lesions. The period of discomfort and virus shedding in acute HSV-2 lesions is reduced by oral acyclovir. Acyclovir does not prevent subsequent recurrence. Intravenous acyclovir is the treatment of choice in encephalitis and disseminated infection.

Prevention

Active cases should be isolated from babies and the immunosuppressed. Health care personnel with herpetic whitlows or other active lesions should not work with infants or the immunosuppressed. Sexual activity should be avoided in acute HSV-2 disease. An experimental vaccine is being evaluated.

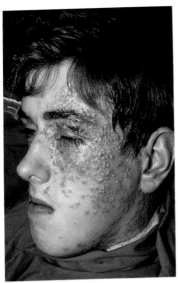

Fig. 34 Kaposi's varicelliform eruption (eczema herpeticum).

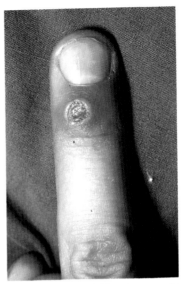

Fig. 35 Herpetic whitlow (surgeon's finger).

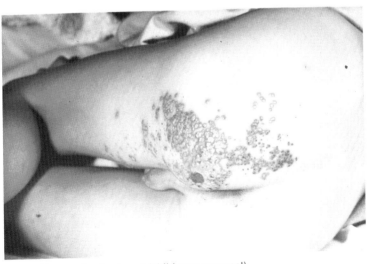

Fig. 36 Herpes simplex type 2 (child, non-venereal).

8 | Smallpox

Aetiology

Variola major and variola minor: the smallpox viruses.

Incidence

Global eradication was achieved in 1977.

Pathogenesis

Transmitted by airborne droplet emission from pharynx of, and direct contact with, active cases. Invasion of the upper respiratory tract was followed by virus multiplication in reticuloendothelial tissue, viraemia and prodromal illness.

Clinical features

The incubation period of about 12 d was followed by pyrexia, malaise, backache and headache and, occasionally, by a maculopapular rash. This prodromal illness was followed 2–3 d later by the major rash, which appeared peripherally and then spread over the body (Figs 37 & 38). Initially macular, the rash became vesicular (round, deep set lesions commonly showing central umbilication) and then pustular (Fig. 39). Death resulted from severe toxaemia, complicating pneumonitis, bacterial pneumonia or sudden cardiovascular collapse. Mortality was commonly 30% or more. Variola minor (alastrim) was a milder form with a lesser systemic upset, sparse rash and a mortality of less than 1%.

Treatment

Vaccination and hyperimmune globulin were used to prevent or modify the disease after contact.

Prevention

Global eradication was achieved by vaccinial vaccination utilising a heat-stable, freeze-dried vaccine and mass case-finding, contact tracing and 'ring' vaccination techniques. Vaccination had potential complications (p. 25).

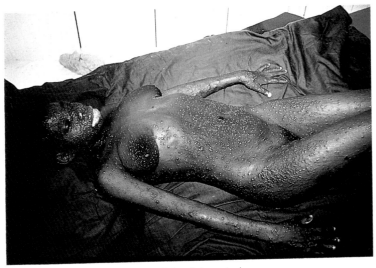

Fig. 37 Generalised smallpox rash (variola major).

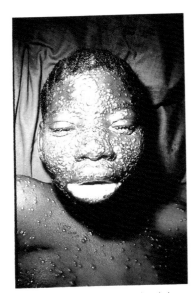

Fig. 38 Facial appearance (variola major).

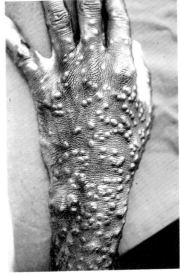

Fig. 39 Detail of rash: deep set lesions with early central umbilification.

9 | Vaccinial Vaccination Complications

Aetiology

Vaccinia virus: a large pox virus.

Incidence

Global smallpox eradication has left little requirement for vaccination. Vaccination complications are therefore rare.

Features of vaccination

After primary vaccination a vesicle appears in 3–5 d and develops into an umbilicated pustule, reaching maximum size in 9–10 d. It then scabs and scars. Immunity against smallpox lasts some years.

Complications

1. Accidental inoculation: of other sites by contact with vaccination site (Fig. 40).
2. Calf lymph hypersensitivity (Fig. 41).
3. Generalised vaccinia: an extensive toxic vesicular rash with significant mortality usually occurs in immunosuppressed individuals.
4. Eczema vaccinatum (Figs 42 & 43): occurs in atopic patients, localised to affected skin.
5. Vaccinia gangrenosa: is an uncontrolled ulceration spreading from the primary inoculation site usually in agammaglobulinaemic patients.
6. Post-vaccinial encephalitis: a rare occurrence 10–13 d after vaccination.
7. Vaccination in pregnancy may cause still-birth or generalised vaccinia of the fetus.

Treatment

Antivaccinial immune globulin or beta-thiosemicarbazone given early may be effective in generalised vaccinia, eczema vaccinatum and vaccinia gangrenosa.

Prevention

Vaccination is now only recommended for selected health care and laboratory workers. Pregnant, atopic or immunosuppressed patients must not be vaccinated nor come in contact with recently vaccinated individuals.

INFECTIOUS DISEASES

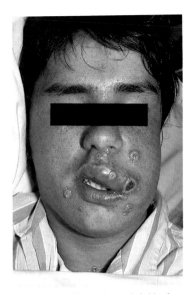

Fig. 40 Umbilicated vaccinial lesions after accidental contact.

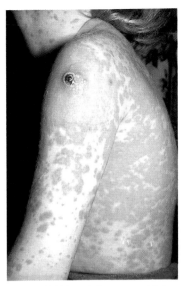

Fig. 41 Calf lymph hypersensitivity reaction: primary vaccination.

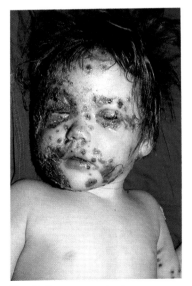

Fig. 42 Eczema vaccinatum.

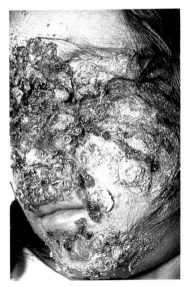

Fig. 43 Secondarily infected eczema vaccinatum.

10 | Orf

Aetiology

Orf virus: an ovoid paravaccinia virus.

Incidence

A common world-wide zoonosis of sheep and goats in which it causes watery papillomatous lesions on the mucosae and conjunctivae. Man is infected by direct occupational contact with the animal, most commonly during spring lambing. Now rare in the UK due to preventative veterinary vaccines.

Pathogenesis

A nodule appears at the site of contact where virus enters through a laceration or abrasion of the skin. A vesiculobulbous hyperplastic mass develops, usually without further spread.

Clinical features

Shepherds are infected at lambing time but shearers, abbatoir workers and veterinary surgeons can also catch orf. Exposed surfaces such as hands, forearms or the face are usually affected. An irritating but pain-free nodule develops, enlarges and has a gelatinous appearance (Fig. 44). It may be incised (wrongly) but no material expressed. Healing (Fig. 45) takes some weeks but there is no scarring. Secondary bacterial cellulitis or lymphangitis may occur. Erythema multiforme is an occasional complication. Virus can be isolated from the lesion and demonstrated by electron microscopy.

Treatment

No specific treatment is available. Erythromycin or cloxacillin are effective for secondary bacterial infection. The lesion should not be incised.

Prevention

Gloves should be worn when handling infected animals. Isolation of patients is unnecessary. An effective ovine vaccine is now available which prevents enzootic disease in sheep.

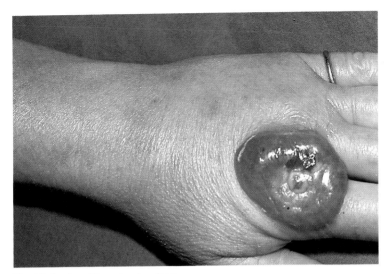

Fig. 44 Acute orf in a shepherdess.

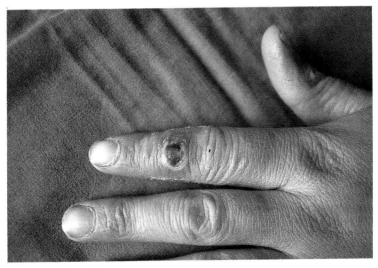

Fig. 45 Healing orf.

11 | Herpangina

Aetiology

Coxsackie viruses types 1–6, 8, 10 (commonly) and other types (rare).

Incidence

Predominantly sporadic, but subject to minor epidemic fluctuations. May be accompanied by an upsurge of viral meningitis, enteritis and infantile febrile episodes due to the same epidemic type. A significant proportion of infections are asymptomatic or trivial.

Pathogenesis

Spread occurs mainly by the faecal–oral route and, less commonly, via airborne droplet emission, usually amongst young schoolchildren who transmit infection to older siblings and parents.

Clinical features

Herpangina is characterised by fever, moderate systemic toxaemia and ulcerative pharyngitis. The onset is acute and resolution may take up to a week. Fluctuant pyrexia is present for the initial few days accompanied by ulcers of the palatal pillars, posterior soft palate and uvula (and less commonly of the tonsils and posterior aspect of the tongue) (Fig. 46). The ulcers are 1–5 mm in size, are covered by necrotic slough, and spare the anterior of the mouth — in contrast with herpes simplex stomatitis and Stevens–Johnson syndrome. There is no accompanying rash. Diagnosis is primarily clinical but may be supported by virus isolation from throat and stool.

Treatment

No specific therapy is available and antibiotics are not indicated. Symptomatic relief may be obtained with aspirin gargles.

Prevention

Not notifiable: isolation not necessary. No specific preventative measures are available.

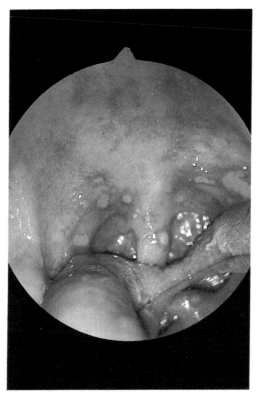
Fig. 46 Herpangina: ulceration of fauces.

12 | Hand, Foot and Mouth Disease

Aetiology

Coxsackie virus A16 (occasionally A5 or A10).

Incidence

This unusual clinical manifestation of enteroviral activity is associated with clusters of clinical cases when infection is widespread in the community. Virus is often isolated from asymptomatic family contacts. World-wide distribution.

Pathogenesis

Spreads primarily by faecal–oral transmission and probably also by the airborne droplet route. Viraemia is followed by a typically distributed skin rash with oral lesions.

Clinical features

The incubation period is 3–7 d and is followed by the appearance of bright red spots or small vesicles on the buccal mucosa, which ulcerate and then heal within 7–10 d. These spare the back of the throat and affect mainly the lips, tongue, and inside of the cheeks and palate. A sparse, painless rash of the hands and feet affects the lateral aspects of fingers and toes but also involves the palm and soles. The skin lesions (Figs 47 & 48) vary from red macules to small vesicles, containing milky fluid, and bullae which may ulcerate and heal 7–10 d later. In infancy the buttocks may be affected. In children, mild fever and malaise are common but adults usually have little systemic upset. Virus can be isolated by tissue culture or material from oral and skin lesions. Specific serum antibodies show a diagnostic rise in titre.

Treatment

Symptomatic. Antibiotics are not indicated.

Prevention

Good hygiene — although by the time of diagnosis other household members will already be infected, whether symptomatic or not.

INFECTIOUS DISEASES

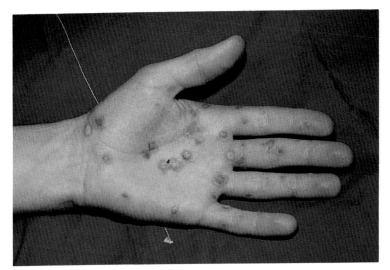

Fig. 47 Palmar vesicles.

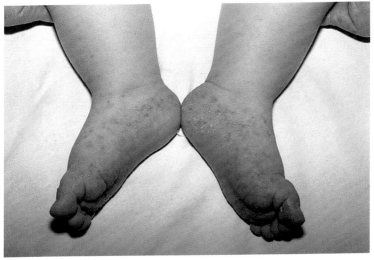

Fig. 48 Milky vesicles on feet.

Infectious Mononucleosis (IM) (1)

Aetiology

Epstein–Barr virus (EBV), a herpes virus.

Incidence

World-wide distribution causing glandular fever (Europe and N. America). EBV is also associated with Burkitt's lymphoma (Africa) and nasopharyngeal carcinoma (Far East). Inapparent infection is common, especially in lower socio-economic groups. Clinical glandular fever is most often seen among affluent adolescents.

Pathogenesis

Close contact and kissing facilitate transmission of EBV from saliva. The individual transmitting the illness is often asymptomatic. After oropharyngeal invasion, virus infects B-lymphocytes which form heterophile antibody. Some B-cells are transformed and EBV-containing B-cells continue to replicate. Next, killer T-cells destroy some EBV infected B-cells and suppressor T-cells limit B-cell transformation. The T-cell response causes the lymph node and splenic enlargement, anginose sore throat and the characteristic atypical lymphocytes seen in the peripheral blood. Later a long lasting balance occurs between infected B-cells and killer T-cells. If transformed B-cells proliferate, in the absence of T-cells, or if virus overwhelms B-cells causing agammaglobulinaemia, fulminating disease results.

Clinical features

The incubation period of about 4–8 wk is followed by an illness of 2–3 wk duration, characterised by sore throat, malaise, fever, splenomegaly and generalised tender lymphadenopathy. Pus and pseudomembrane cover the tonsils (Fig. 49) but resolve in 1–2 wk. Cervical lymphadenopathy and periorbital oedema are prominent (Figs 50 & 52), and palatal petechiae are typical (Fig. 51). Hepatomegaly and

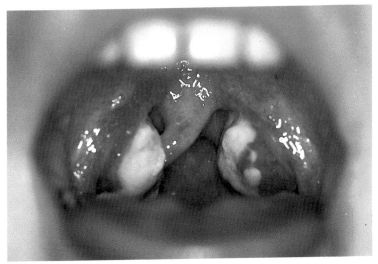

Fig. 49 Anginose pharyngitis with wash-leather exudate.

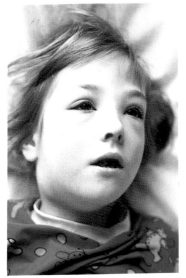

Fig. 50 Facial oedema and cervical lymphadenopathy.

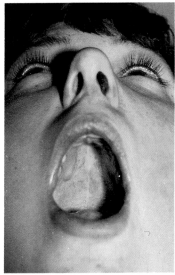

Fig. 51 Palatal petechiae.

Infectious Mononucleosis (IM) (2)

Clinical features (contd)

mild jaundice, and a pink macular rash occur less commonly (Figs 53 & 54). Life-long immunity is conferred. A number of diagnostic investigations are available. Atypical mononuclear cells are present in the peripheral blood and the Monospot slide test and Paul Bunnell test for IgG antibodies are positive. Rising titres of EBV specific IgM and IgG antibodies can be demonstrated.

Complications

Splenic rupture, airways obstruction, blood dyscrasias or CNS complications occasionally prove fatal. Haemolysis, thrombocytopenia, pneumonitis, encephalitis, meningitis, post-infectious polyneuropathy, lymphoma and myocarditis may occur. Administration of ampicillin or amoxycillin typically causes a maculopapular skin rash in IM (Fig. 53). Transient depression is a frequent sequel.

Treatment

Adequate rest is important. Prednisolone or emergency tracheostomy are sometimes required for severe pharyngeal oedema causing incipient respiratory obstruction. Superimposed streptococcal infection is treated with penicillin or erythromycin. Ampicillin or amoxycillin are contraindicated.

Prevention

No active or passive immunisation is available. Strict isolation is not necessary.

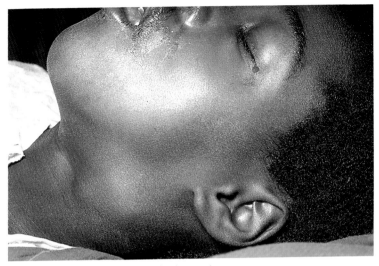

Fig. 52 Cervical lymphadenopathy (severe).

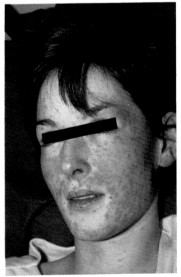

Fig. 53 Jaundice and ampicillin rash.

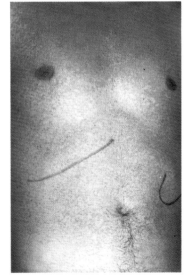

Fig. 54 Rash and hepato-splenomegaly.

14 | Toxoplasmosis

Aetiology

Toxoplasma gondii, an intracellular protozoon parasite.

Incidence

Usually an asymptomatic infection, rarely producing acute disease. Congenital infection occurs in 0.1% of live births.

Pathogenesis

A zoonosis, primarily a disease of cats but also of intermediates such as birds. Acquired by ingestion of oocysts, commonly from kitten faeces, or by airborne droplet transmission. The parasite disseminates in reticuloendothelial and other tissues with secondary spread of trophozoites. Latent infection and transplacental fetal spread may follow.

Clinical features

1. *Acquired disease*. Mononucleosis syndrome characterised by fever, atypical mononucleosis lymphadenopathy and splenomegaly is common. Choroidoretinitis (Figs 55 & 56) and encephalitis are rare.
2. *Congenital disease*.
   a. *Disseminated:* jaundice, lymphadenopathy, splenomegaly, choroidoretinitis.
   b. *CNS disease:* hydrocephalus, convulsions, intracranial calcification (Fig. 57). Perinatal mortality 10–20%.
3. *Opportunistic disease*. Reactivation of latent infection in immunosuppressed patients may cause severe encephalitis.

Toxoplasmosis is diagnosed serologically (Sabin–Feldman dye test and IgM titres).

Treatment

Severe ocular or CNS involvement is treated with pyrimethamine plus a sulphonamide for 3–4 wk. Additional steroid therapy is useful in choroidoretinitis.

Prevention

Not notifiable: isolation not necessary. No adequate control measures are available.

INFECTIOUS DISEASES

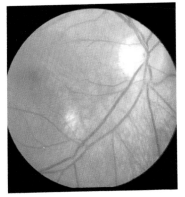

Fig. 55 Acute choroidoretinitis.

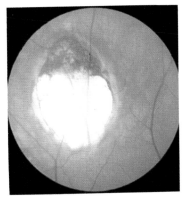

Fig. 56 Healed choroidoretinitis.

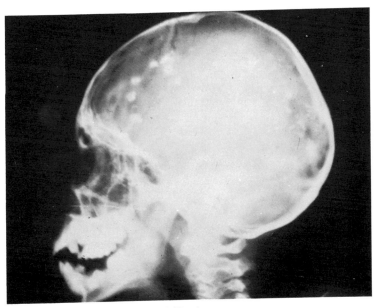

Fig. 57 Congenital intracranial calcification.

15 | Cytomegalovirus (CMV) Infection

Aetiology

Cytomegalovirus: a DNA containing herpes virus.

Incidence

World-wide distribution. Most infections are subclinical but many symptomatic intra-uterine, neonatal and adult acquired infections occur. The peak incidence is between the ages of 1 and 2 yr and 15–30 yr.

Pathogenesis

Spreads by airborne droplet transmission from infected nasopharyngeal secretions. Transplacental infection may arise from primary maternal infection or from reactivation of latent virus infection during pregnancy. Perinatal infection results from maternal cervical infection. Infected infants excrete virus in the urine for months. CMV infected cells swell and show intranuclear and intracytoplasmic inclusions. Nuclear chromatin is pushed to the edge of the cell giving an 'owl's eye' appearance.

Clinical features

1. *Congenital CMV disease* (Fig. 58): results in choroidoretinitis, hepatosplenomegaly, jaundice, rash, microcephaly and deafness.
2. *Acquired CMV disease:* is clinically indistinguishable from infectious mononucleosis although membranous pharyngitis is uncommon. In immunosuppressed patients primary or reactivational CMV causes severe pneumonitis with a mortality of 50%. Choroidoretinitis may occur.

Diagnosis is established by virus isolation from tissues, urine and saliva and a rising antibody titre. An atypical lymphocytosis is usually found in peripheral blood.

Treatment

Symptomatic treatment only. Acyclovir is ineffective in neonatal infection and in pneumonitis in immunocompromised patients.

Prevention

Vaccine development is being undertaken.

INFECTIOUS DISEASES

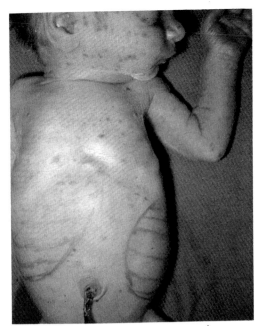
Fig. 58 Congenital rash and hepatomegaly.

16 | Virus Hepatitis

Aetiology

Hepatitis A (HAV), B (HBV) and non-A, non-B (NANBV) viruses.

Incidence

World-wide distribution. HAV affects the young and is often subclinical. HBV is infrequent in the West, except in homosexuals and addicts, but is common in the tropics. NANBV occurs sporadically.

Pathogenesis

HAV is transmitted by the faecal–oral route from cases; HBV by contact, sexual and parenteral routes from cases and carriers; and NANBV via blood products and direct contact. Neonatal HBV infection is acquired from carrier mothers. Viral hepatitis causes centrilobular hepatocyte necrosis and portal inflammation.

Clinical features

The incubation periods are: HAV 15–40 d, HBV 50–140 d, NANBV 30–160 d. Illness starts with malaise, nausea, vomiting, mild fever and abdominal discomfort. Arthralgia may herald hepatitis B. A week later, after the onset of dark urine and pale stools, jaundice appears (Fig. 59). Evidence of addiction may be seen in HBV infections (Fig. 60). Altered consciousness, a flapping tremor and fetor hepaticus precede complicating coma (Fig. 61). Infections with HBV and NANBV can progress to chronic hepatitis. The diagnosis of acute hepatitis is confirmed by an HAV-specific IgM response, demonstration of HBV surface antigen (Fig. 62) or by exclusion (NANBV).

Treatment

Bed rest and symptomatic measures.

Prevention

Notification, isolation, screening of blood donors for HB$_s$Ag and active HBV immunisation. Hyperimmune anti-HBV immunoglobulin for postexposure prophylaxis, neonates of HB$_s$Ag carrier mothers and human normal immunoglobulin for travellers to endemic HAV areas.

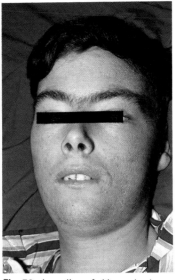

Fig. 59 Jaundice of skin and sclerae.

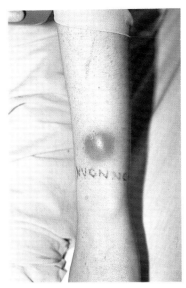

Fig. 60 Addict's arm: tattoo, needle track and abscess.

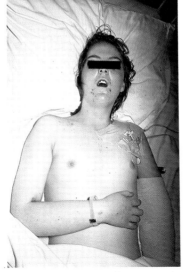

Fig. 61 Terminal hepatic coma: note bruising.

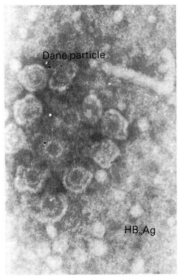

Fig. 62 Electron micrograph: HB$_s$Ag and Dane particles (whole virus) in serum.

17 | Leptospirosis

Aetiology

Leptospira icterohaemorrhagiae, L. hebdomadis and *L. canicola:* pathogenic spirochaetes.

Incidence

About 100 cases/year in the UK, similar order of frequency in Europe, commoner in Tropics.

Pathogenesis

Zoonosis transmitted from reservoirs in rats (*L. icterohaemorrhagiae*), cattle (*L. hebdomadis*) and dogs or pigs (*L. canicola*), usually by skin contact with urine of infected animals. Produces multisystem disease including hepatitis, nephritis, meningitis, coagulopathies and immune-complex disease.

Clinical features

1. Weil's disease (*L. icterohaemorrhagiae*): prodromal headache, myalgia, pyrexia, rigors and prostration are followed a week later by hepatitis and nephritis, and haemorrhage caused by disseminated intravascular coagulation. Haemorrhagic herpes labialis and subconjunctival haemorrhages are often present (Fig. 63).
2. *L. hebdomadis* infection: milder form of Weil's disease, often with lymphocytic meningitis.
3. Canicola fever (*L. canicola*): prodromal syndrome less severe than Weil's disease, followed by lymphocytic meningitis. Jaundice is uncommon. Leptospiral agglutination tests are usually diagnostic. Urine cultures may be helpful.

Complications

Hepatorenal failure causes death in 10% of patients with Weil's disease. Transverse myelitis, uveitis and myopericarditis may occur.

Treatment

Benzyl penicillin or tetracycline are effective only if given in the prodromal phase.

Prevention

Notification: isolation not necessary. Veterinary vaccines. Hygiene in farms, abbatoirs and kennels.

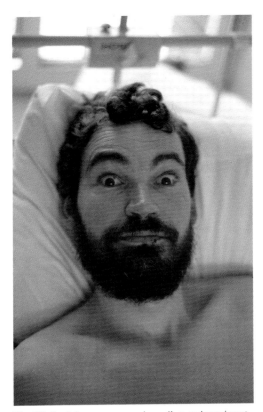

Fig. 63 Facial appearance: jaundice, subconjunctival haemorrhage, haemorrhagic herpes labialis.

18 | Staphylococcal Infection (1)

Aetiology

Coagulase-positive *Staphylococcus aureus*. The skin commensal *Staph. albus* (*epidermidis*) may infect prostheses and ventriculoatrial shunts, and is also associated with urinary tract infection in women.

Incidence

World-wide. Severe opportunistic infections may occur in immunocompromised patients and diabetics.

Pathogenesis

Pathogenic staphylococci are often carried on skin or anterior nares and may cause endogenous or exogenous infection by invasion, toxin production or both. Staphylococci enter skin breaches or hair follicles causing local sepsis, polymorphonuclear leucocytosis and pus formation. Invasion of bronchial mucosa devitalised by influenza leads to staphylococcal pneumonia. Superficial infections (impetigo, boils, carbuncles and deeper cellulitis) may result in bacteraemia with endocarditis and widespread sepsis. Toxin production or absorption of preformed toxin can cause enterotoxin food poisoning, exotoxin induced toxic (tampon) shock syndrome and exfoliatin induced toxic epidermal necrolysis (TEN).

Clinical features

1. Skin infections: impetigo (Fig. 64) affects only the superficial epidermis and is highly infectious. A boil (Fig. 65) is a tender, inflamed infected hair follicle from which pus may discharge spontaneouly. Coalescence of infected follicles may result in a carbuncle. In cellulitis (Fig. 66) deeper tissues are infected.
2. Bacteraemia results from superficial or deep sepsis or from direct injection of staphylococci by drug addicts. In 50% endocarditis occurs with widespread septic emboli to brain, lungs, skin (Fig. 67) and kidneys. Staphylococcal pneumonia commonly results in empyema and lung abscesses, notably in children with mucoviscidosis.

INFECTIOUS DISEASES

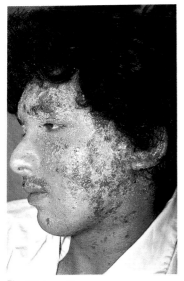

Fig. 64 Impetigo.

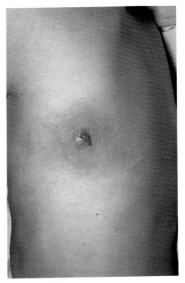

Fig. 65 Boil exuding yellow pus.

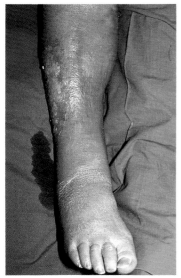

Fig. 66 Cellulitis with epidermal necrosis.

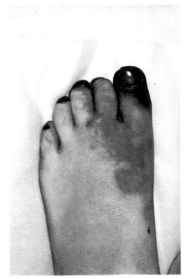

Fig. 67 Septic embolic gangrene in endocarditis.

Clinical features (contd)

3. Toxin-induced disease: staphylococcal food poisoning starts 1–2 h after eating preformed enterotoxin with profuse vomiting and prostration but without diarrhoea. Exotoxin-A induced toxic or tampon shock is characterised by fever, hypotension and rash. Staphylococci are found high in the vagina but rarely on blood culture. In TEN, infants with scalded skin syndrome (Ritter's disease: Figs 68 & 69) or children with Lyell's syndrome (Fig. 70) develop painful erythematous shearing of superficial epidermal bullae. TEN also occurs in immunocompromised adults (Fig. 71). Staphylococci can usually be isolated from affected sites except in TEN and food poisoning.

Treatment

Superficial skin sepsis is treated with dressings, poulticing or surgical drainage. Deeper or systemic infection requires urgent parenteral chemotherapy with flucloxacillin, fusidic acid or clindamycin. IV fluids, oxygen, physiotherapy and surgical drainage of septic arthritis, lung abscess and empyema may be necessary. Prosthetic valve replacement is frequently required in endocarditis.

Prevention

Scrupulous hand washing; asepsis in surgery and in the care of neonates; cleansing traumatic wounds; isolation and/or treatment of staphylococcal carriers; improved food hygiene.

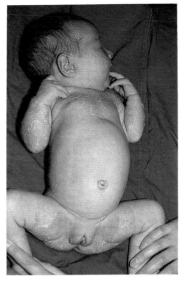

Fig. 68 Ritter's Disease.

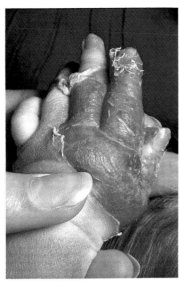

Fig. 69 Ritter's Disease

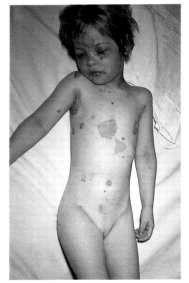

Fig. 70 Lyell's syndrome.

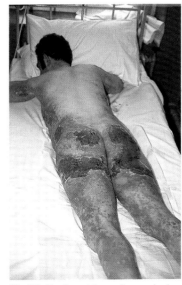

Fig. 71 Toxic epidermal necrolysis (lymphoma patient)

19 | Osteomyelitis (OM)

Aetiology

Staphylococcus aureus causes 80% of cases of OM, most of the remainder being due to *Strep. pyogenes, H. influenzae* and, less commonly, enterobacteria. Salmonella, pseudomonas and tuberculous OM are rare in UK.

Incidence

Staphylococcal OM is commonest in males aged between 3 and 10 yr. Distribution is world-wide but commoner in warm climates and amongst those with sickle cell disease and diabetes mellitus. Prosthetic hip joints may be infected.

Pathogenesis

During bacteraemia which is often asymptomatic or trivial, staphylococci settle in metaphyses or sites of bone injury. About 60–70% of staphylococcal OM occurs in the easily traumatised lower limbs. Local inflammation leads to pus formation, periosteal elevation and bone necrosis secondary to septic thrombosis. X-ray changes take several weeks to develop.

Clinical features

A history of injury may be given. The onset is sudden with fever, rigors and exquisitely tender local inflammation in the bone or joint. Untreated, septic sinus formation (Fig. 72), bone necrosis leading to sequestrum formation (Fig. 73) and pathological fracture occur. The causal organism can be identified in blood (50–60% positive), bone biopsy and joint fluid cultures. Leucocytosis is usual. X-ray changes take several weeks to develop.

Treatment

Antibiotics are given for 4–6 wk. Clindamycin, fusidic acid and flucloxacillin give good results in staphylococcal OM. Other organisms are treated according to their sensitivities. Surgical drainage is required in 50%.

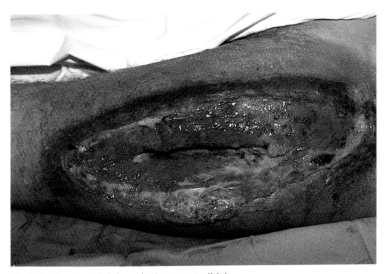

Fig. 72 Sinus in thigh (surgical osteomyelitis).

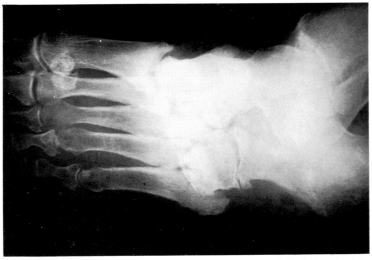

Fig. 73 Disorganised tarsus (osteomyelitis complicating diabetic foot ulcer).

20 | Infections with *Streptococcus pyogenes* (1)

Aetiology

Beta-haemolytic streptococci: classified by cell wall carbohydrates into Lancefield's groups and by T-proteins into Griffith's types.

Incidence

World-wide distribution. Pyoderma mainly affects children with poor hygiene in the tropics. Scarlet fever, rheumatic fever and post-streptococcal glomerulonephritis are now rare except in the developing world.

Pathogenesis

Both asymptomatic carriers and those with active disease spread group A infection by airborne droplet transmission causing pharyngitis, follicular tonsillitis and cervical adenitis. Skin infection is facilitated by hyaluronidase which assists pyoderma to spread and involve deeper tissues, producing erysipelas and cellulitis. Erythema nodosum, and later rheumatic fever and glomerulonephritis, are immunological reactions to streptococcal infection. Neonates acquire group B streptococci from the birth canal and develop septicaemia (within 5 d) or later septicaemia and meningitis.

Clinical features

1. *Erysipelas:* streptococcal invasion of the skin may result in a butterfly facial rash, (Figs 74 & 75) or a spreading eruption on the legs characterised by a red, swollen, painful epidermal lesion with a well demarcated raised edge. Bullae may form.
2. *Pyoderma* (Fig. 76): type 49 streptococci cause epidemics of skin sepsis with yellow crusts (with or without nephritis).
3. *Ascending lymphangitis* (Fig. 77): represents tender red inflamed lymph channels draining a streptococcal infection.

INFECTIOUS DISEASES

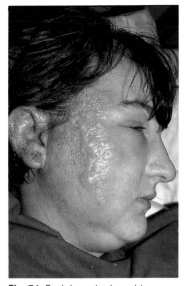

Fig. 74 Facial erysipelas with superficial bullae.

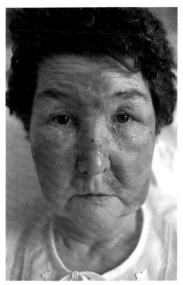

Fig. 75 Healing erysipelas: note raised edge.

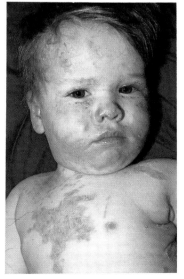

Fig. 76 Streptococcal pyoderma.

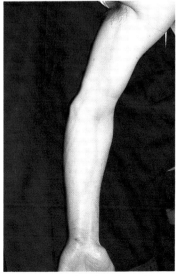

Fig. 77 Ascending lymphangitis from wound at wrist.

Infections with *Streptococcus pyogenes* (2)

4. *Pharyngitis, tonsillitis and quinsy:* after 2–4 d incubation, sore throat, fever, tachycardia and malaise are associated with pharyngitis or follicular tonsillitis (Fig. 78) and cervical adenitis. A bulging peritonsillar abscess (quinsy) may follow (Fig. 79). More rarely, suppurative adenitis, sinusitis, otitis media or mastoiditis develop. Viral pharyngitis, glandular fever and diphtheria must be differentiated.
5. *Ludwig's angina* (Fig. 80): infection in the submandibular space. May follow dental extraction in immunocompromised patients and can cause airways obstruction.
6. *Henoch-Schoenlein purpura* (Fig. 81): affecting the buttocks and legs, and associated with arthritis and intestinal colic or bleeding, is commonly related to streptococcal infection.
7. *Erythema nodosum* (Fig. 82): may complicate many acute infections, especially streptococcal or tuberculous, and sarcoidosis or drug therapy. Tender, red, raised lesions develop on the shins or elbows (p. 97).
8. *Rheumatic fever:* begins 2–3 wk after a streptococcal infection with fever, tachycardia, cardiac arrythmias and murmurs, flitting large joint arthralgia, subcutaneous nodules and rashes like erythema marginatum (Fig. 83). Two major or one major and two minor criteria with evidence of recent streptococcal disease confirm the diagnosis.
Major: carditis, polyarthritis, chorea, erythema marginatum, subcutaneous nodules.
Minor: fever, joint pain, high ESR or C-reactive protein, leucocytosis, prolonged P-R interval, past history of rheumatic fever.

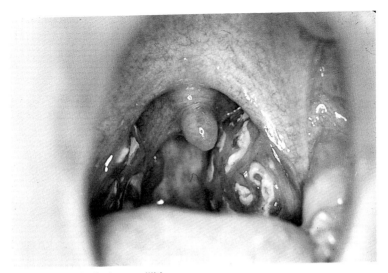

Fig. 78 Acute follicular tonsillitis.

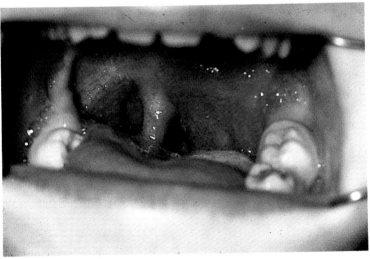

Fig. 79 Acute peritonsillar abscess (quinsy) with trismus.

Infections with *Streptococcus pyogenes* (3)

Clinical features
(contd)

9. *Glomerulonephritis:* group A, type 12 or, during an epidemic of pyoderma, type 49 infections may be followed by fever, oedema, hypertension and oliguria, proteinuria, haematuria and casts in the urine.
Diagnosis of streptococcal infections requires isolation of streptococci from the throat, saliva or skin or demonstration of a rising ASO titre. A polymorphonuclear leucocytosis and high ESR are usual.

Treatment

Penicillin-G is advised initially but may be followed by oral penicillin-V as the condition improves. Erythromycin is recommended for penicillin-allergic patients. To prevent recurrences of rheumatic fever, penicillin-V (or erythromycin) prophylaxis is used. High dose amoxycillin immediately before dental surgery prevents *Strep. viridans* endocarditis. Specific treatment is necessary for cardiac failure and arrythmias in rheumatic fever and renal failure in glomerulonephritis.

Prevention

Hospitalised patients should be isolated for 48–72 h, until chemotherapy renders them non-infectious.

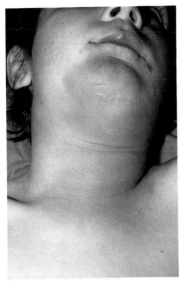

Fig. 80 Ludwig's angina.

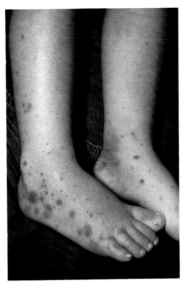

Fig. 81 Henoch–Schoenlein purpura.

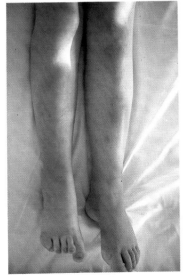

Fig. 82 Erythema nodosum.

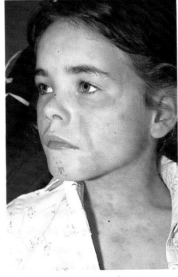

Fig. 83 Erythema marginatum.

21 | Scarlet Fever

Aetiology

Beta-haemolytic streptococci of Lancefield's Group A elaborating erythrogenic toxin.

Incidence

World-wide distribution. Previously common in the developed countries, it is now rarely seen and is a milder disease than formerly.

Pathogenesis

Both asymptomatic carriers and clinical cases disseminate streptococci, usually in airborne droplets. Wounds may also be a portal of entry. Secondary sepsis of ears, nose and peritonsillar region can occur.

Clinical features

The incubation period of 2–4 d is followed by the sudden onset of sore throat, fever, headache and often vomiting, contrasting with the slower onset of diphtheria and glandular fever. The tonsils are red and flecked with pus, and peritonsillar inflammation and oedema may develop, associated with tender cervical adenitis. The tongue is initially furred and white (Fig. 84) and later smooth and red (Fig. 86). The rash consists of a scarlet blush (Fig. 85) with a punctate erythema which spares the circumoral region (Fig. 84). It peels after a few days (Fig. 86). Peripheral skin peeling is often marked on the palms and soles (Fig. 87). Streptococci isolated from throat swabs, a polymorphonuclear leucocytosis and a rising ASO titre confirm the diagnosis.

Treatment

Penicillin-G followed by penicillin-V or, in penicillin-allergic patients, erythromycin.

Prevention

Isolation is desirable in the acute phase.

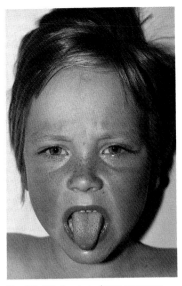

Fig. 84 White strawberry tongue with circumoral pallor.

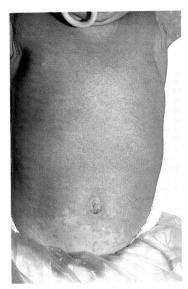

Fig. 85 Punctate erythema.

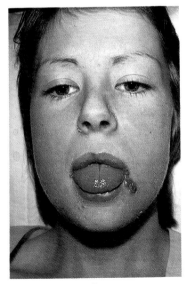

Fig. 86 Red strawberry tongue, perinasal peeling and herpes febrilis.

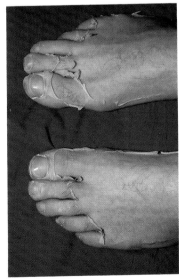

Fig. 87 Peripheral superficial skin peeling.

22 | Anthrax

Aetiology
: *Bacillus anthracis*, a Gram-positive sporing bacillus.

Incidence
: Rare in UK but commoner in Europe and elsewhere due to animal enzootic disease.

Pathogenesis
: A zoonosis acquired from contact with active cases amongst domestic mammals, including sheep, cattle and pigs, and (in UK) with imported spore-infected hides, hair and unsterilised bone meal. Spores may be directly inoculated into the skin (cutaneous anthrax), inhaled (pulmonary anthrax) or, more rarely, ingested (intestinal anthrax).

Clinical features
: 1. *Cutaneous anthrax* (most common): a local papule at the site of inoculation develops into an ulcerated, necrotic, dark-centred eschar (malignant pustule: Figs 89 & 91), associated with extensive oedema (Figs 88 & 90), regional adenitis and fever. Complicating septicaemia is uncommon.
  2. *Pulmonary anthrax* (uncommon): severe disseminated haemorrhagic bronchopneumonia. Complicating septicaemia is common.
  3. *Intestinal anthrax* (rare): varies from mild enteritis to a severe dysenteric illness.
  Diagnosis is confirmed by isolation of *B. anthracis* from pustule, sputum, stools or CSF.

Complications
: 1. Haemorrhagic pleuropericarditis.
  2. Haemorrhagic meningitis.

Treatment
: Benzyl penicillin (10–20 megaunits/d) for 7 d. Antiserum therapy is no longer used.

Prevention
: Notifiable: strict isolation is necessary. A vaccine is available for those at risk of occupational exposure, e.g. professional gardeners (bone meal) and those handling imported hair and hides.

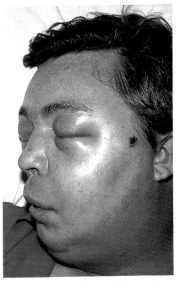

Fig. 88 Facial anthrax with massive oedema (gardener).

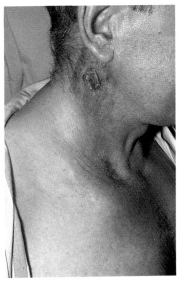

Fig. 89 Cervical eschar (bone meal worker)

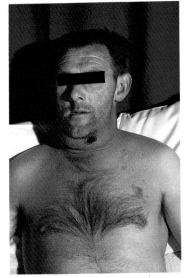

Fig. 90 Eschar and oedema of neck and chest wall (farmer).

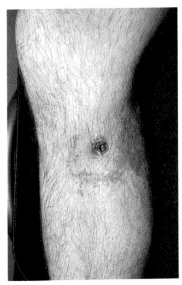

Fig. 91 Eschar on leg (bone meal worker).

23 | Diphtheria

Aetiology

Toxigenic *Corynebacterium diphtheriae,* a Gram positive bacillus.

Incidence

World-wide distribution: diphtheria is rare where there is a high rate of immunisation.

Pathogenesis

Airborne droplet transmission from cases. *C. diphtheriae* multiplies in the upper airways and forms an adherent membrane of bacteria, WBC and necrotic tissue. There is associated oedema of the neck. Laryngeal obstruction can occur in infants. Absorption of a potent toxin causes later cardiac and neurological complications.

Clinical features

The incubation period of 2–4 d is followed by fever, disproportionate tachycardia, malaise, headache and symptoms at the site of invasion — nose, tonsils, pharynx or larnyx (Figs 92 & 93). Typical adherent membrane appears on mucosa (Fig. 93), associated with lymphadenopathy and surrounding oedema (bull-neck appearance). Stridor may be present in infants with laryngeal diphtheria. Diphtheria toxin causes cardiac arrhythmias, conduction defects and failure 1–3 wk after onset and, later, peripheral neuropathies. These include palatal, ocular, diaphragmatic (phrenic nerve) and late onset limb pareses, 3–10 wk after onset.

Treatment

10 000–60 000 units of antitoxin are given intravenously if a diluted intradermal test dose shows no significant reaction. Benzyl penicillin or erythromycin should be prescribed.
Tracheostomy is occasionally indicated.

Prevention

Notifiable: strict isolation is mandatory. Routine immunisation (toxoid vaccine) is given in infancy. Carriers should be treated with erythromycin.

INFECTIOUS DISEASES

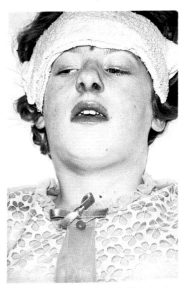

Fig. 92 Nasopharyngeal diphtheria with bloody discharge and bull neck.

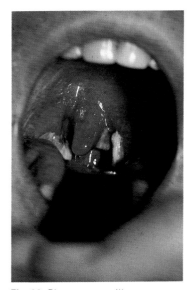

Fig. 93 Pharyngotonsillar diphtheria: note adherent membrane with curled edge.

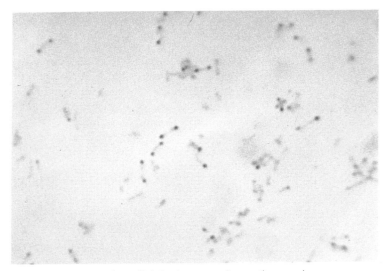

Fig. 94 *Corynebacterium diphtheriae:* metachromatic granules.

24 | Tetanus

Aetiology

Clostridium tetani, an anaerobic, Gram-positive sporing bacillus.

Incidence

World-wide distribution: commoner where there is no immunisation, and in farming communities.

Pathogenesis

Cl. tetani is an environmental organism which is introduced into deep traumatic anaerobic wounds or into the umbilical stump in neonates. Vegetative multiplication and toxin elaboration follows. Two toxins are produced:
1. *Tetanolysin:* which causes labile hypertension, arrhythmias, vasoconstriction and sweating.
2. *Tetanospasmin:* which fixes to nuclei of motor nerves and neuromuscular end-plates causing muscle spasm.

Clinical features

The incubation period is usually 5–14 d, dependant on the size and site of the inoculum. Cephalic tetanus has a short incubation and poor prognosis. The onset of muscular spasm and rigidity is insidious and characterised by trismus, risus sardonicus and, later, opisthotonos (Fig. 95a). Spasms are triggered by noise, lights or movement. Consciousness and sensation are unimpaired. Respiratory arrest or asphyxia may occur. Neonatal tetanus begins 3–10 d after birth and has a very poor prognosis (Fig. 95b).

Treatment

Mainly supportive. Muscular spasms should be controlled with intravenous diazepam. Therapeutic paralysis and IPPV are infrequently required. Human tetanus immunoglobulin (30 iu/kg; iu = international units) and benzyl penicillin should be administered.

Prevention

Traumatic wounds must be thoroughly cleansed. Toxoid vaccine and human tetanus immunoglobulin should be given as required. All infants should be routinely immunised.

INFECTIOUS DISEASES

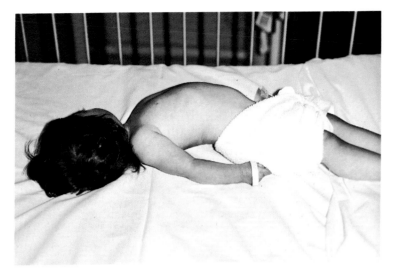

Fig. 95a Tetanic spasm (opisthotonos).

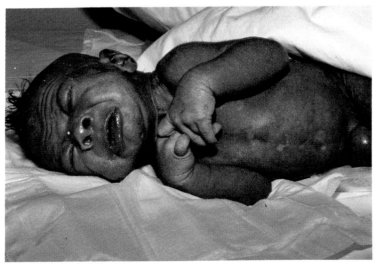

Fig. 95b Neonatal tetanus (wrinkled brow and risus sardonicus).

25 | Enteric (Typhoid and Paratyphoid) Fevers

Aetiology	*Salmonella typhi, paratyphi* A and B
Incidence	World-wide distribution: commoner in warmer climates and where poor hygiene/sanitation prevail. Typhoid in the UK is usually imported from Asia.
Pathogenesis	Faecal-oral transmission via contact and contamination of water and food. Ingested *S. typhi* not killed by gastric acid, enter the ileum, invade lymphatics and multiply in the reticulo-endothelial (RE) system. Subsequent bacteraemia and re-invasion of the gut is responsible for the clinical illness.
Clinical features	The initial bacteraemic phase, which lasts for about a week, is characterised by a step-wise rise in fever, relative bradycardia, constipation, splenomegaly, increasing confusion and, less commonly, a pink, macular (rose spot) truncal rash (Fig. 96). Untreated, the patient then deteriorates with increasing toxaemia, dehydration, a maintained fever, and abdominal cramps and diarrhoea (Fig. 97). Recovery usually commences in the third week but relapse and intestinal perforation or haemorrhage may occur. Diagnosis is confirmed by blood and stool cultures, and a specific 'O' antibody response in the Widal test. Stools often remain positive for several weeks but permanent carriage occurs in less than 5%.
Treatment	The antibiotics of choice are chloramphenicol, co-trimoxazole and amoxycillin. Intravenous chemotherapy and fluid replacement may be needed. Prolonged co-trimoxazole therapy eradicates gut carriage in up to 50%: cholecystectomy cures 75%.
Prevention	Notifiable: strict isolation is necessary. Good hygiene/sewage disposal and clean water supplies are essential. Monovalent typhoid vaccine gives partial protection for 3 yr.

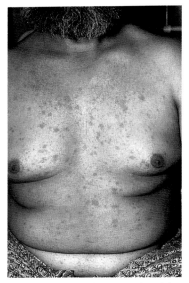

Fig. 96 Extensive 'rose spot' rash in paratyphoid A.

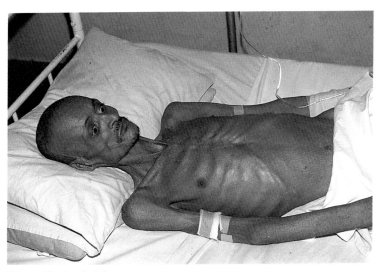

Fig. 97 The 'typhoid' state.

26 | Infantile Gastroenteritis (1)

Aetiology

Usually viral, due to rotavirus (30%) or other small round viruses (astroviruses and caliciviruses) and enteroviruses, but may also be due to enteropathogenic *Escherichia coli* (EPEC) serotypes (0111, 0128, 0142, etc.) or *Salmonella, Shigella* or *Campylobacter* species. In 40% no aetiological agent is identified.

Incidence

Diarrhoeal illness is amongst the commonest causes of morbidity and hospital admission in infants in the UK. It is responsible for up to 25% of total infant morbidity in developing countries and in many such areas is the commonest cause of death in infancy.

Pathogenesis

Acquisition follows faecal–oral transmission from acute cases (viruses, shigella, EPEC), via foodstuffs or milk/water (salmonellosis, campylobacteriosis) or from carriers (salmonellosis). Enteritis is caused by either gut wall invasion and inflammation (e.g. shigellosis and salmonellosis), adherence and cytotoxicity (e.g. rotavirus and EPEC enteritis), or invasion of the gut wall plus enterotoxin production (e.g. campylobacterosis).

Clinical features

The cardinal features are diarrhoea and vomiting, which vary from trivial to profuse. Blood staining of faeces is more typical of invasive disease due to bacteria, especially shigellosis and campylobacterosis. Fluid loss may cause dehydration, hypovolaemia and hypotension (Figs 98, 99 & 100). Excoriation of the buttocks and perineum may occur (Fig. 101). Bacteraemia may accompany salmonellosis and EPEC enteritis

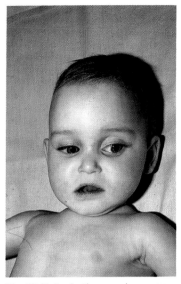

Fig. 98 Dehydration: sunken eyes, corrugated axillary folds and dry mouth.

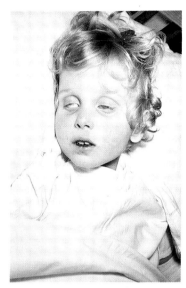

Fig. 99 Severe dehydration.

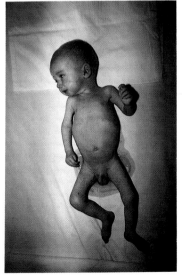

Fig. 100 Dehydrated infant; clear fluid stool after glucose/electrolyte feed.

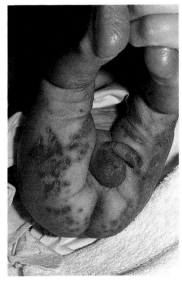

Fig. 101 Excoriation of buttocks and perineum.

Clinical features (contd)

but is uncommon with other bacterial diarrhoeas in the UK. Diagnosis requires stool and, where relevant, blood cultures. Enteropathogenic viruses in stools may be demonstrated by electron microscopy (Fig. 102).

Compli-cations

1. *Hypernatraemia:* was most commonly associated with the use of hypertonic milk feeds (no longer marketed) during early disease and was associated, in severe cases, with intracranial sinus thrombosis, secondary cerebral oedema causing focal or generalised convulsions and neurological defects, and renal thrombosis/necrosis (Fig. 103).
2. *Acute colitis:* can follow salmonellosis or campylobacterosis but is unusual in children.
3. *Lactose intolerance:* transient secondary disaccharidase deficiency can follow rotavirus or EPEC enteritis. It usually settles within 2 mth, and requires substitution of non-lactose containing milks.

Treatment

Rehydration using oral or parenteral glucose-electrolyte solutions, e.g. ½ strength Hartmanns solution or Dioralyte, followed by reintroduction of graduated, increasing strength milk feeds over 3–4 d. Antibiotics are contra-indicated except in bacteraemic infants.

Prevention

Many forms notifiable (e.g. salmonellosis). Hospitalised cases must be strictly isolated. General preventative measures include food hygiene precautions, aseptic preparation of milk feeds, adequate cooking of contaminated meats, e.g. poultry, encouragement of breast feeding and, notably in developing countries, the provision of clean water supplies and effective sanitation. Rotavirus and other vaccines are under development.

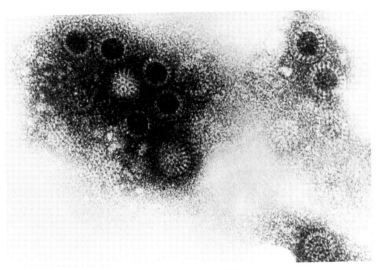

Fig. 102 Electron micrograph of rotavirus particles.

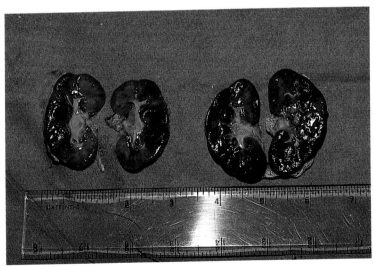

Fig. 103 Bilateral renal thrombosis in dehydrated neonate.

27 | Pseudomembranous Colitis

Aetiology

Enterotoxin producing *Clostridium difficile*, a Gram-positive sporing anaerobe.

Incidence

Rare but may occur in sub-epidemic form in surgical wards. Affects up to 3% of patients receiving clindamycin.

Pathogenesis

Colonic overgrowth of *Cl. difficile* induced by antibiotic exposure, followed by toxin production and mucosal damage typified by summit lesions on colonic mucosa (Fig. 104), glandular disruption, epithelial necrosis and focal inflammation. Macroscopic colonic pseudomembranes are present (Fig. 105). Most commonly follows broad spectrum penicillin and cephalosporin exposure but classically associated with clindamycin. The source of *Cl. difficile* may be hospital cross-infection.

Clinical features

1. *Mild:* slight persistent diarrhoea, self-limiting within 2 wk in 80%.
2. *Severe:* frequent bloody diarrhoea with abdominal and rectal tenesmus associated with fever and dehydration, which may progress to toxic dilatation (Fig. 106), perforation of colon and death. Can present during treatment or for several weeks thereafter.

Diagnosis is substantiated by sigmoidoscopy, rectal biopsy and examination of stools for *Cl. difficile* and enterotoxin.

Treatment

Vancomycin 125 mg, 8-hourly, by mouth for 5 d. Response is usually rapid but up to 10% of patients relapse.

Prevention

Not notifiable: known cases must be isolated to prevent cross colonisation of other patients. Instruments and endoscopes used rectally should be sterilised with sporicidal disinfectants.

INFECTIOUS DISEASES

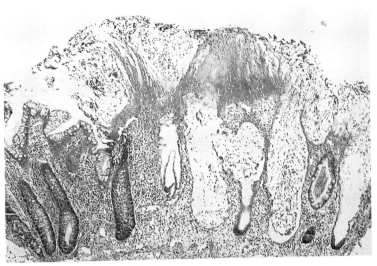

Fig. 104 Histology: summit lesion.

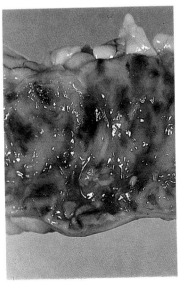

Fig. 105 Colonic pseudomembranes.

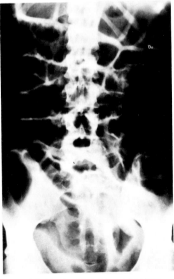

Fig. 106 Toxic dilatation of colon (precolectomy).

Aetiology

Neisseria meningitidis: a Gram-negative diplococcus. Epidemics are due to types A, B and C and sporadic cases are usually caused by types B, W135 and other serotypes.

Incidence

Epidemic fluctuation: about 1000 sporadic cases per year in the UK. Secondary cases may occur in close family and nursery school contacts.

Pathogenesis

Spread occurs via airborne droplet transmission from nasopharynx of cases and carriers. Subsequent fulminating bacteraemia or subacute bacteraemia and meningitis commonly follow, but many acquire asymptomatic nasopharyngeal carriage. In acute cases endotoxin release from intact *N. meningitidis* causes antibody-independent complement activation, shock, disseminated intravascular coagulation and generalised Schwartzman reaction (capillary damage, thrombosis and haemorrhage into skin and adrenals). Immune complex deposition disease may cause arthritis.

Clinical features

1. *Fulminating meningococcaemia:* overwhelming shock, petechiae and ecchymoses (Figs 107, 108, 109 & 110), and adrenal infarction (Fig. 111) (Waterhouse–Friderichsen syndrome); death usually occurs within 6–18 h (Fig. 112). Commonest in infants.
2. *Bacterial meningitis:* severe toxaemia, meningeal irritation and petechial rash associated with a polymorphonuclear CSF pleocytosis (plus low CSF sugar and elevated protein). Usually fatal within 48–72 h if untreated. Commoner in older children and young adults.
3. *Recurrent meningitis:* associated with antibody and late-acting complement component deficiencies (rare).
4. *Pneumonia:* uncommon.

Diagnosis is established by isolation of *N. meningitidis* from CSF and blood cultures.

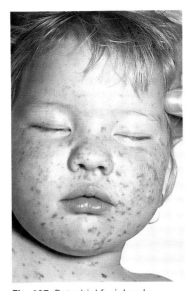

Fig. 107 Petechial facial rash.

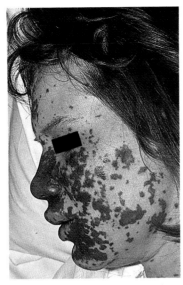

Fig. 108 Ecchymotic facial rash (late stage).

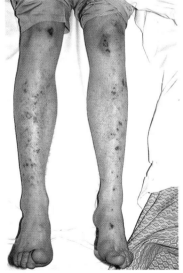

Fig. 109 Haemorrhagic rash (adult with meningitis).

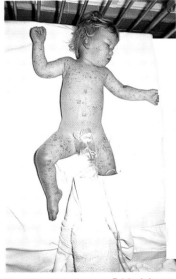

Fig. 110 Waterhouse–Friderichsen syndrome.

**Compli-
cations**

Immune complex arthritis and pericarditis can arise 1 wk or more after onset. Extensive skin necrosis may follow ecchymotic haemorrhage.

Treatment

Intravenous benzyl penicillin (100 000–200 000 iu kg/d) for 7 d. Intrathecal therapy is unnecessary. Chloramphenicol should be used for penicillin-allergic patients. Steroids (for acute adrenal insufficiency) and heparin (for DIC) are of no benefit.

Prevention

Notifiable: strict isolation is necessary, but cases amongst hospital contacts are extremely rare.
1. *Chemoprophylaxis:* close family and nursery school contacts should receive rifampicin (5 mg/kg, 12-hourly) plus, in adults, minocycline (100 mg, 12-hourly) for 2 d. Secondary cases are most likely to occur within 24 h of the index case: chemoprophylaxis should therefore be started immediately.
2. *Immunoprophylaxis:* a vaccine is available for types A and C but is not in general use. It may be used for control of epidemics or individual protection of contacts (chemoprophylaxis preferred).

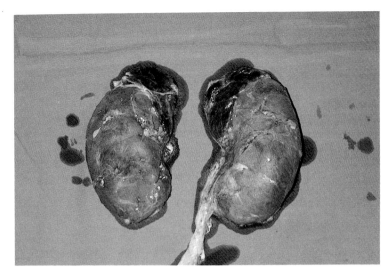

Fig. 111 Bilateral haemorrhagic adrenal infarction.

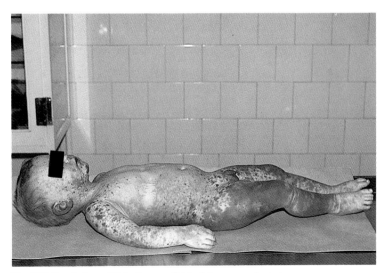

Fig. 112 Death from Waterhouse–Friderichsen syndrome.

29 | Bacterial Meningitis

Aetiology

N. meningitidis, Strept. pneumoniae and *H. influenzae.*

Incidence

2000 cases/yr in the UK: *N. meningitidis* 50%

Pathogenesis

Strept. pneumoniae — usually endogenous. May invade meninges via blood stream, sinuses, middle ear infections or basal fractures. *H. influenzae* (Pittman type B) — an exogenous infection acquired from carriers of the virulent serotype. *N. meningitidis* (p.73). Pathology is characterised by acute inflammatory infiltration of meninges and ependyma of ventricles.

Clinical features

A severe, acute onset illness, characterised within 24–48 h by high fever, headache, neck stiffness (Fig. 113), photobia, vomiting and confusion. Focal CNS signs and coma indicate a poor prognosis. The meningococcal rash (p.74) distinguishes this from other forms. Diagnosis is established by CSF examination (polymorph pleocytosis, low sugar) and isolation of the pathogen from CSF and blood cultures.

Complications

1. Persistent fever: often due to drugs.
2. Intracranial abscess (rare).
3. Sterile subdural effusions (rare).
4. CNS abnormalities: decerebrate rigidity (Fig. 114), hydrocephalus, deafness, epilepsy.
5. Immune-complex arthritis (meningococcal).
6. Septic arthritis (pneumococcal or meningococcal).

Treatment

Meningococcal and pneumococcal meningitis: benzyl penicillin 100 000 iu/kg/d for 10 d. *H. influenzae* and undiagnosed bacterial meningitis: chloramphenicol 50–100 mg kg/d (10 d). Reduce dose for neonates.

Prevention

Notification and isolation of meningococcal infection. Vaccines not generally available.

INFECTIOUS DISEASES

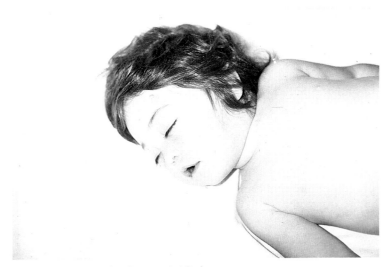

Fig. 113 Neck retraction (severe rigidity).

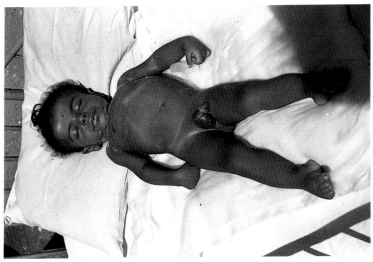

Fig. 114 Decerebrate state (*H. influenzae* meningitis).

30 | Viral Meningitis

Aetiology

Enteroviruses (echovirus, Coxsackie virus, poliovirus) and mumps virus.

Incidence

Epidemic fluctuations in incidence, enteroviruses in most summers and mumps every 3–4 yr. High incidence of asymptomatic infection.

Pathogenesis

Enteroviruses spread via faecal–oral route, most commonly in young children who transmit infection to older family contacts. Mumps infection spreads by droplet airborne transmission from active cases. Both cause lymphocytic meningitis with minimal brain and spinal parenchymal inflammation.

Clinical features

1. Enteroviruses cause a mild prodromal febrile URTI or enteritis followed by recrudescent fever, positional headache, neck and spinal rigidity (Fig. 115), photophobia, vomiting and, in some, a maculopapular rash (Fig. 116) and pharyngitis or conjunctivitis. The patient is usually not very ill.
2. Mumps meningitis causes similar signs of meningeal irritation, usually preceded by salivary gland involvement (p. 9).

Complications

Echo and Coxsackie viruses rarely cause an ascending paralysis similar to poliomyelitis. Mumps may be complicated by orchitis, oophoritis, pancreatitis or arthritis.

Treatment

Analgesia and several days bed rest are required.

Prevention

Poliovirus infections are notifiable: all cases require strict isolation. Poliovaccine is type specific and has no protective effect against other enteroviruses. Echo and Coxsackie virus vaccines are not available. Mumps vaccine is routinely available in the USA.

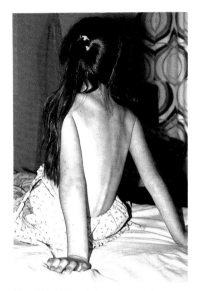

Fig. 115 Tripod sign of spinal rigidity.

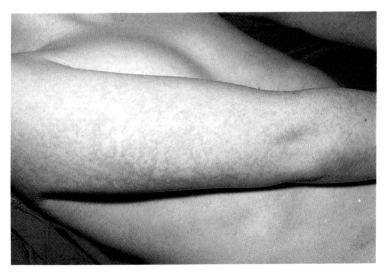

Fig. 116 Enteroviral rash.

31 | Primary Tuberculosis (1)

Aetiology

Mycobacterium tuberculosis (human and bovine).

Incidence

Rare in UK, even amongst high risk immigrant groups. Usually seen in children.

Pathogenesis

Airborne droplet transmission from active pulmonary cases. Inhalation is followed by formation of sub-pleural (Ghon) focus and hilar gland involvement (primary complex) which usually heals but may rupture into bronchus, pleura or pulmonary vessels followed by local, pleural, pericardial, bronchial or haematogenous spread.

Clinical features and complications

1. Asymptomatic infection with healing: Mantoux becomes +ve in 6−8 wk. Primary hilar gland(s) may be obvious on chest X-ray (Fig. 117). Later reactivation may occur (see point 5). Primary infection may be associated with immunological hypersensitivity phenomena including erythema nodosum (see p. 97) and phlyctenular conjunctivitis.
2. Tuberculous pleural effusion: secondary to rupture into pleura, can fill the hemithorax (Fig. 118).
3. Miliary tuberculosis: miliary pulmonary infiltration and widespread dissemination and foci of infection including tuberculous meningitis. The chest X-ray usually has a characteristic 'snowstorm' appearance (Fig. 119). Choroidal tubercles may be present (Fig. 120).

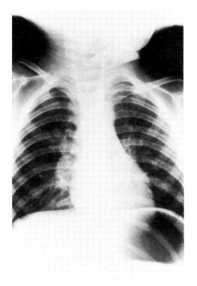

Fig. 117 Primary tuberculous gland at right hilum.

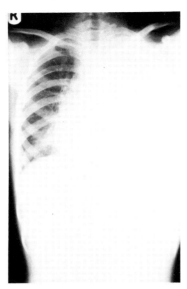

Fig. 118 Primary tuberculous pleural effusion.

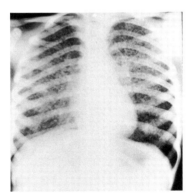

Fig. 119 Miliary tuberculosis (snowstorm appearance).

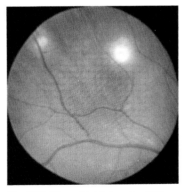

Fig. 120 Choroidal tubercles (TB meningitis).

Clinical features and complications (contd)

4. Tuberculous bronchopneumonia: either localised to a segment (epituberculosis) or widespread throughout both lungs (Fig. 121). Can result in rapid weight loss and death within months (galloping consumption).
5. Late complications: tuberculous pericarditis, tuberculous osteitis and arthritis (after 5−10 yr) (Fig. 122), renal tuberculosis (after 10−15 yr), reactivation of pulmonary disease in adulthood (Fig. 123). Late pericardial involvement may cause calcification of pericardium and constrictive pericarditis.

Treatment

Triple therapy: rifampicin, ethambutol and isoniazid. Pyrizinamide is often added in patients with tuberculous meningitis. Severely ill children and many with tuberculous meningitis require steroid therapy. Asymptomatic infections in contacts require active triple therapy (if x-ray abnormal) or prophylactic isoniazid (if X-ray remains normal).

Prevention

Notifiable: isolation is necessary for several weeks until effective chemotherapy has rendered respiratory secretions and urine non-infective. All close contacts should be screened to detect the source of infection (usually a family member) and other early cases, notably amongst siblings. Those converting to Mantoux positivity require follow-up chest X-ray and, in many cases, anti-tuberculous chemotherapy (see above). BCG vaccination is routinely administered to early teenage children in the UK but is given neonatally in high risk immigrant groups.

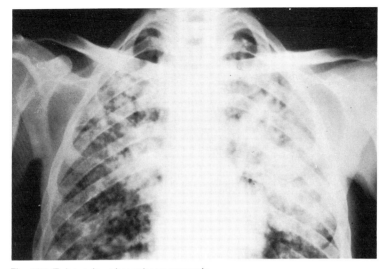

Fig. 121 Tuberculous bronchopneumonia.

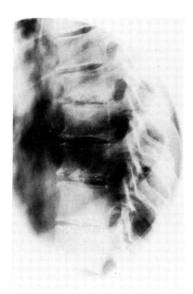

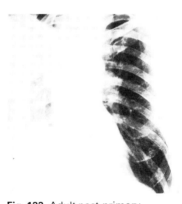

Fig. 123 Adult post-primary pulmonary tuberculosis (healed fibrotic disease).

Fig. 122 Tuberculous spondylitis: note erosion of vertebral bodies (Pott's disease).

32 | Pertussis (Whooping Cough)

Aetiology

Bordetella pertussis, a Gram-negative bacillus.

Incidence

Sporadic disease, subject to epidemic variation every 3–5 yr.

Pathogenesis

Airborne droplet transmission from active cases. Inflammatory bronchitis is accompanied by mucosal necrosis and mucus hypersecretion, peribronchial infiltration and, in severe cases, plugging of airways and absorption collapse.

Clinical features

The incubation period of about 5–10 d is followed by upper respiratory catarrh, lasting for about a week. The paroxysmal cough then develops, accompanied by terminal inspiratory whoop and persists for several weeks. Cough may cause cyanosis, vomiting and transient apnoea. Chest examination is usually normal between paroxysms.

Complications

1. *Respiratory:* secondary bacterial bronchopneumonia and lung abscess, segmental/lobar/pulmonary collapse (Figs 124 & 125), bronchiectasis.
2. *Neurological:* a rare encephalopathy is characterised by convulsions, coma and progressive CNS signs.
3. *Pressure-related:* paroxysmal cough may cause subconjunctival haemorrhage (Fig. 126), skin petechiae, herniae and rectal prolapse.

Treatment

Oral erythromycin (30 mg kg/d for 5 d) given within 1 wk of onset may attenuate severity.

Prevention

Notifiable: hospitalised cases require strict isolation. Polyvalent whole cell derived agglutinogen vaccine gives 95% protection. Erythromycin given to contacts within 5 d may prevent disease.

INFECTIOUS DISEASES

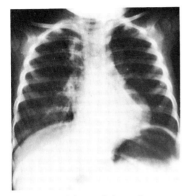

Fig. 124 Left lower lobe collapse: shadow behind the heart.

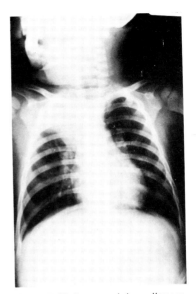

Fig. 125 Right upper lobe collapse: right apex.

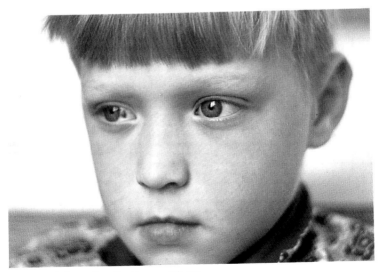

Fig. 126 Sub-conjunctival haemorrhage.

33 | Acute Croup and Bronchiolitis

Aetiology

Para-influenza (croup) and respiratory syncitial virus (bronchiolitis).

Incidence

Acute croup usually affects children from 3 to 36 mth and bronchiolitis infants less than 3 mth. Both are cold weather illnesses and are distributed world-wide.

Pathogenesis

Spread by airborne droplet transmission from active cases. In croup, oedema and inflammatory narrowing of upper airways result in stridor and hoarseness. Bronchiolitis, is associated with necrosis, paralysis of cilia and mucus plugging of terminal airways.

Clinical features

1. *Croup:* mild fever and coryza are followed by hoarseness, barking cough, inspiratory stridor and increasing distress always worse at night.
2. *Bronchiolitis:* the baby may be afebrile but is distressed with nasal flare, tracheal tug, cough, subcostal and intercostal recession, crepitations and rhonchi. Dyspnoea prevents feeding, leading to dehydration.

The chest X-ray may be clear or show peribronchitis (Fig. 127) or bronchopneumonia. Cardiac failure may occur in very young infants. Diagnosis is achieved by examination of nasopharyngeal secretions by FAT and tissue culture.

Treatment

Severely ill babies are treated with oxygenated, humidified air. Severe croup requires use of IV hydrocortisone to clear the oedematous airway. Bronchiolitic babies may need antibiotics, such as amoxycillin, bronchodilators and IV fluids.

Prevention

No vaccines are currently available.

INFECTIOUS DISEASES

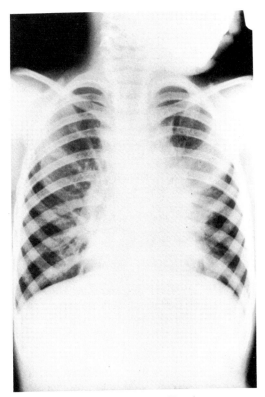

Fig. 127 Diffuse peribronchial infiltration.

34 | Legionnaires' Disease

Aetiology

Legionella pneumophila and other species: small Gram-negative coccobacilli.

Incidence

May account for 3–5% of atypical pneumonias. Sporadic incidence is intermixed with common-source outbreaks in hotels and hospitals.

Pathogenesis

Legionellae are environmental organisms which become established in air-conditioning and shower systems. Aerosols probably account for inhalational acquisition by most patients. Multisystem infection follows, associated with severe bronchiolopneumonitis. Renal failure and CNS involvement are rare but can be severe.

Clinical features

The incubation period of 2–10 d is followed by malaise, fever, myalgia, rigors, headache and diarrhoea. Mental confusion is prominent. Failure of empirical penicillin therapy is typical. Dry cough develops but other respiratory signs, may be minimal. Several days later, crepitations may be heard but consolidation is often absent. Chest X-ray shows lobar or diffuse infiltration (Fig. 128). Serological tests (IFAT) confirm the diagnosis. Untreated disease may last 2–3 wk.

Complications

Renal and respiratory failure, and cerebellar ataxia may occur. The mortality is about 10%.

Treatment

I.v. erythromycin is the drug of choice. Rifampicin is added in non-responding patients.

Prevention

Case-to-case transmission does not occur: isolation is not necessary. Infected water systems should be adequately and, if necessary, repeatedly chlorinated. Notification may be required by some authorities.

INFECTIOUS DISEASES

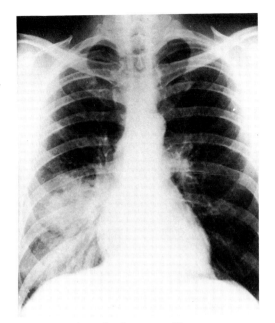

Fig. 128 Legionnaires' pneumonitis

35 | Atypical Pneumonia

Aetiology	*Mycoplasma pneumoniae, Chlamydia psittaci* and *Coxiella burnetii*.
Incidence	*M. pneumoniae* pneumonia is common in younger people. Psittacosis is acquired from birds (parrots, budgies and pigeons) and is seen in fanciers and handlers. Q-fever is a disease of sheep, goats and cattle, occasionally seen in vets and farmers.
Pathogenesis	The pathogen is usually inhaled: by droplet emission from active cases (*M. pneumoniae*) or aerosol/dust from contaminated environments (psittacosis/Q-fever). All cause pneumonitis.
Clinical features	These diseases have an incubation period of 1–3 wk and a subacute onset. Prodromal features may include fever, rigors, myalgia/arthralgia, anorexia, vomiting and pharyngitis. These are followed by dry cough, associated with a mild pneumonitis which can be patchy, multifocal or perihilar (Figs 129 & 130). Occasionally severe pneumonia can occur. Signs of consolidation are often absent. The illness may last for 2–3 wk and the diagnosis is established serologically.
Complications	1. *Mycoplasma pneumonitis:* arthritis, haemolysis, encephalitis and Stevens–Johnson syndrome (p. 99). 2. *Q-fever:* endocarditis 3. *Psittacosis:* renal failure, encephalitis, endocarditis and DIC.
Treatment	Erythromycin is the drug of choice for *M. pneumoniae* pneumonia. Tetracycline is preferred for Q-fever and psittacosis.
Prevention	Avoidance of exposure and hygiene measures in bird and animal husbandry. Experimental vaccines are not generally applicable. Routine isolation of active cases is not necessary.

INFECTIOUS DISEASES

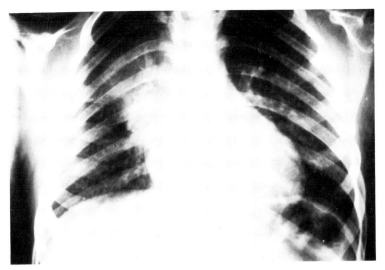

Fig. 129 *Mycoplasma pneumoniae* pneumonia.

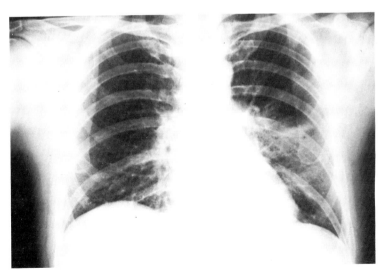

Fig. 130 Psittacosis pneumonitis (hazy left mid-zone infiltration).

36 | Bacterial Pneumonia

Aetiology

Lobar pneumonia is usually caused by *Strept. pneumoniae* and bronchopneumonia additionally by *Staph. aureus*, and *H. influenzae*. Primary Gram-negative pneumonia is rare.

Incidence

Usually sporadic but hospital outbreaks may be caused by Gram-negative pathogens.

Pathogenesis

Pneumococcal pneumonia is an endogenous infection. *Staph. aureus* infections may complicate influenza and other viral URTI. *H. influenzae* pneumonia occurs in children or in chronic bronchitics. Gram-negative bacilli, e.g *Esch. coli.*; *Klebsiella* spp. and *Ps. aeruginosa*, cause opportunistic infections particularly in granulocytopenic cancer patients. *Klebsiella* spp. pneumonia may occur in the elderly.

Clinical features

Range from localised consolidation, toxaemia and fever to severe bacteraemic disease with local and systemic complications, and shock (notably in Gram-negative infections). Chest X-ray demonstrates lobar consolidation (Fig. 131) or multifocal opacification.

Complications

Include lung abscess (p. 95), empyema, bacteraemia, meningitis (usually Gram-negative infections) and other metastatic disease.

Treatment

Strept. pneumoniae — benzyl penicillin; *H. influenzae* — amoxycillin; *Staph. aureus* — cloxacillin plus fusidic acid; *Gram-negative infections* — gentamicin plus, in compromised patients, azlocillin; *severe undiagnosed pneumonia* — gentamicin plus erythromycin.

Prevention

Polyvalent pneumococcal vaccine (Pneumovax) for predisposed patients, e.g. sickle cell disease, post-splenectomy and severe bronchitics.

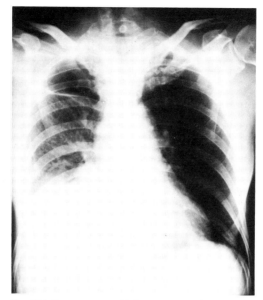

Fig. 131 Pneumococcal lobar pneumonia.

37 | Lung Abscess

Aetiology

Strept. pneumoniae (post-pneumonic), oral anaerobes (post-aspiration), *Staph. aureus* (post-pneumonic), mixed flora (post-embolic abscess).

Incidence

A sporadic endogenous infection.

Pathogenesis

May complicate primary pneumonia (pneumococci, *Staph. aureus* and Gram-negative bacilli), aspiration of oral secretions (comatose or ventilated patients), pulmonary infarction, tricuspid endocarditis (usually *Staph. aureus* in heroin addicts) or lobar collapse.

Clinical features

May present as: a complication of known pneumonia, unexplained fever in comatose or ventilated patients, a recurrence of fever in patients with pulmonary embolism or tricuspid endocarditis, haemoptysis and fever, or pyrexia of unknown origin.
Physical signs can be minimal in the absence of overlying pleurisy or complicating empyema. Foul sputum usually indicates anaerobic infection. Chest X-ray is usually diagnostic (Fig. 132).

Treatment

Prolonged antibiotic courses of 6–8 wk are usually required. Post-pneumonic and aspiration abscess should be treated with benzyl penicillin and metronidazole. Staphylococcal lung abscess requires cloxacillin plus fusidic acid. Complicating empyema must be surgically drained.

Prevention

Important factors include adequate therapy of primary pneumonias, physiotherapy and tracheostomy care of comatose or ventilated patients, and rapid bronchoscopic clearance of obstructed airways.

INFECTIOUS DISEASES

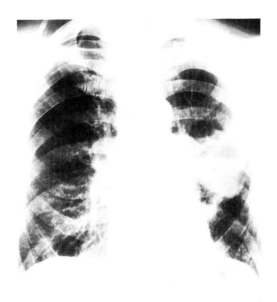

Fig. 132 Post-aspiration lung abscess: fluid level.

38 | Erythema Nodosum

Aetiology

Multiple precipitants including primary tuberculosis, streptococcal disease, intestinal infections, e.g. yersinosis and campylobacteriosis, sarcoidosis, chronic inflammatory bowel disease and many drugs including combined oral contraceptives.

Incidence

Uncommon. Infections are the commonest cause in children; acute sarcoid and contraceptive pill in young women.

Pathogenesis

A non-infective, non-suppurative localised vasculitis caused by an immunologically-mediated reaction to infective or chemical stimuli, or immunologically based disease.

Clinical features

Acutely tender circumscribed erythematous nodules, 1–4 cm diameter, usually confined to anterior surface of legs below knees (Figs 133 & 134). May appear successively for several weeks but usually settle spontaneously within a few weeks if drug or infection related. May persist or recur in sarcoidosis or auto-immune disease. In acute sarcoidosis erythema nodosum is usually associated with arthritis, hilar adenopathy and fever, and occasionally with phlyctenular conjunctivitis and parotitis.

Treatment

Removal of aetiological factor, e.g. cessation of drugs, eradication of infection or treatment of auto-immune disease. If not contra-indicated by aetiology (e.g. infections), steroids can have a beneficial effect.

Prevention

May require isolation, dependant on causation. Avoidance of previously recognised drug precipitants.

INFECTIOUS DISEASES

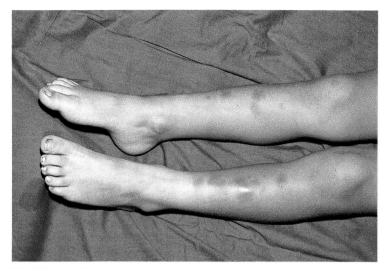

Fig. 133 Early discrete erythema nodosum.

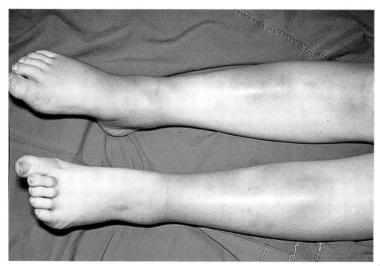

Fig. 134 Late coalescent erythema nodosum.

39 | Stevens-Johnson Syndrome

Aetiology	May complicate therapy with various drugs including sulphonamides and penicillins, and infections caused by herpes simplex, *Mycoplasma pneumoniae* and streptococci.
Incidence	Sporadic and uncommon.
Pathogenesis	Results from immune hypersensitivity mechanisms of uncertain type which cause vasculitis in the skin, mucous membranes and conjunctivae leading to vesiculobullous lesions.
Clinical features	Conjunctival, genital and mucocutaneous lesions of variable severity. Erosive lesions may be found on the lips, buccal mucosa, tongue and genitalia (Figs 135 & 136). Skin lesions are almost invariably present, commonly on the hands and feet, commencing as a multiform eruption subsequently forming vesicles and bullae which may coalesce (Figs 137 & 138). Evolution and regression takes place over 2–3 wk and healing may be accompanied by desquamation, skin pigmentation or superficial scarring.
Complications	Secondary bacterial skin and oral infection is common. Recurrent H. simplex infections may precipitate further episodes of Stevens–Johnson syndrome.
Treatment	Most cases require symptomatic therapy alone. Secondary skin infections may require treatment with flucloxacillin. Precipitating *M. pneumoniae* infections are treated with erythromycin. Steroids are of unproven benefit.
Prevention	Nil presently available. Aetiologically-related drugs must be avoided.

INFECTIOUS DISEASES

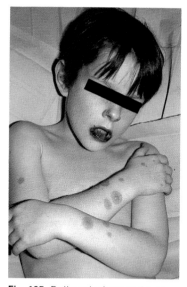

Fig. 135 Bullous lesions and oral ulceration.

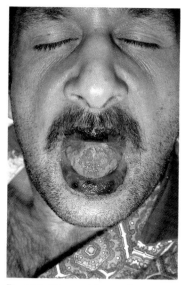

Fig. 136 Ulcers of lips and tongue.

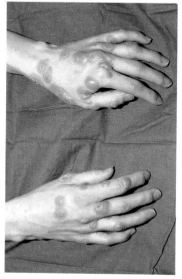

Fig. 137 Vesiculobullous lesions.

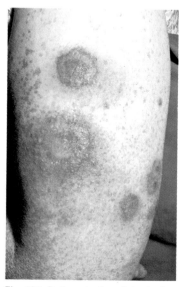

Fig. 138 Bullous lesions (atypical).

40 | Antibiotic Rashes

Aetiology

Many antibiotics cause skin rashes, most notably the penicillins, cephalosporins and sulphonamides. Rashes are less commonly caused by erythromycin, chloramphenicol, clindamycin and tetracyclines and only rarely follow the use of aminoglycosides.

Incidence

The overall incidence is approximately:
1. Penicillins: 2–3% (ampicillin up to 7%).
2. Cephalosporins: 1–2% (10% of penicillin-allergic patients also react to cephalosporins.
3. Sulphonamides (and co-trimoxazole): 5%.

Pathogenesis

Antibiotics may engender immediate hypersensitivity (IgE-mediated) reactions, usually causing urticaria, or delayed reactions both of the serum-sickness (IgG-mediated) type and by other ill understood mechanisms, including induction of sensitised lymphocytes. The reaction can be due to the parent antibiotic, high molecular weight polymers, or breakdown products.

Clinical features

The penicillins, cephalosporins and sulphonamides may all cause urticaria (Fig. 139), morbiliform eruptions (Fig. 140) or erythema multiforme (Fig. 141) and, rarely, Stevens–Johnson syndrome (p. 99).

Complications

Drug rashes are usually transient but may be part of a generalised hypersensitivity reaction.

Treatment

Early treatment of urticaria with antihistamines or corticosteroids may hasten recovery. Antihistamines are also useful for pruritus associated with morbiliform penicillin/cephalosporin rashes. Treatment is otherwise symptomatic.

Prevention

Implicated antibiotics should be avoided in the future.

| INFECTIOUS DISEASES

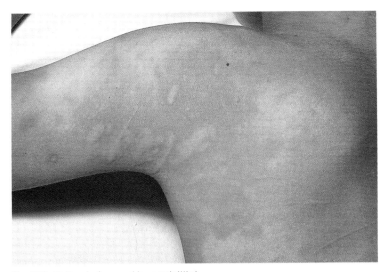

Fig. 139 Urticaria (caused by penicillin).

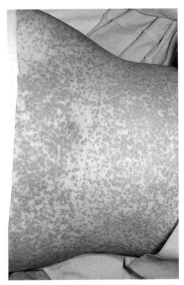

Fig. 140 Morbilliform rash (caused by ampicillin)

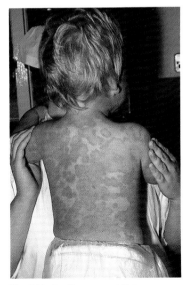

Fig. 141 Erythema multiforme (caused by sulphonamide)

41 | Secondary Syphilis

Aetiology	*Treponema pallidum*, a spirochaete.
Incidence	World-wide distribution: high incidence in homosexuals.
Pathogenesis	Sexually transmitted: man is the only host. The local chancre of acquired syphilis starts 9–90 d after sexual contact and is followed 6 wk to several months later by secondary syphilis. Secondary disease merges into latent endarteritic syphilis in which physical signs are absent but serology, as in secondary syphilis, is positive. Tertiary syphilis causes neurological or cardiovascular disease years later.
Clinical features	Secondary syphilis mimics many skin infections and infestations, including mononucleosis, acute exanthemata, erythema multiforme, condylomata accuminata, alopecia areata and oral or vaginal candidiasis. Macular, maculopapular (Fig. 142) and pustular skin lesions with vesicles last for 1–2 mth. They occur anywhere but mainly on the palms (Fig. 143) and soles. Condylomata lata are non-tender, moist greyish plaques in intertriginous areas, frequently in the perineum. These and mucosal 'snail track' ulcers are highly infectious. Fever, laryngitis, pharyngitis, arthralgia, painless lymphadenopathy and weight loss occur. The diagnosis of secondary syphilis is confirmed by dark ground examination of exudates for *T. pallidum* and positive serology.
Treatment	Intramuscular procaine penicillin 600 000 iu, daily for 10 d. The possibility of a Jarisch–Herxheimer reaction may be covered with corticosteroids.

INFECTIOUS DISEASES

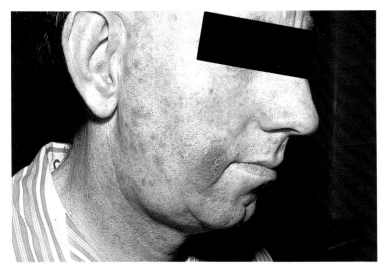

Fig. 142 Papulonodular secondary syphilitic rash.

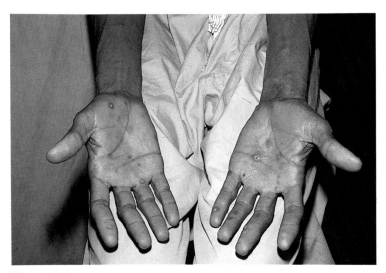

Fig. 143 Palmar lesions in secondary syphilis (in Arab).

42 | Gonococcaemia

Aetiology

Neisseria gonorrhoea, a gram-negative diplococcus.

Incidence

A sporadic complication of genital, anorectal and oropharyngeal gonorrhoea.

Pathogenesis

Occurs as a complicating bacteraemia with organ involvement in patients with gonorrhoea, which in females may be asymptomatic, or, in pharyngeal disease, may be unsuspected.

Clinical features

Initially presents as a pyrexia of unknown origin accompanied by sparse, violaceous macular or vesicular skin lesions (50%) (Figs 144 & 145), or as a pyrexia with organ involvement, most commonly arthritis (80%). Monarticular septic arthritis usually presents a week or more after onset but polyarticular, hypersensitivity-mediated small joint arthritis may present within a few days. Endocarditis is a later, uncommon complication (5%) causing aggressive valvular lesions. Gonococcal meningitis is also uncommon (5%). Diagnosis is established by blood culture and isolation of *N. gonorrhoeae* from endocervical, vaginal, urethral, anorectal and pharyngeal swabs. Concomitant syphilis must be excluded.

Treatment

A 10-d course of high-dose benzyl penicillin is adequate for uncomplicated disease but patients with septic arthritis or endocarditis should receive at least 4–6 wk treatment. Penicillin resistant gonococcaemia may be treated with cefuroxime.

Prevention

Not notifiable: hospitalised cases should be isolated. Routine contact tracing should be undertaken to arrange treatment and prevent secondary disease.

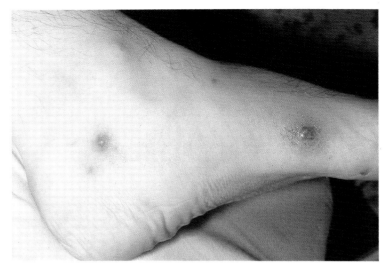

Fig. 144 Violaceous vesicular lesions (iodine self-medication).

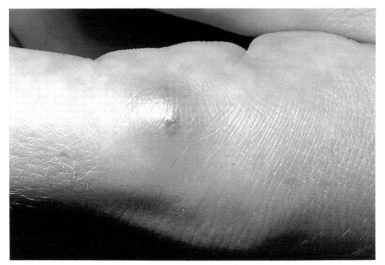

Fig. 145 Papulovesicular lesion.